# DRUGS:

## An Annotated Bibliography and Guide to the Literature

by
**Alfred M. Ajami, Jr.**
in collaboration with
The Sanctuary
Cambridge, Massachusetts

G. K. HALL & CO., 70 LINCOLN STREET, BOSTON, MASS.

1973

**Library of Congress Cataloging in Publication Data**

Ajami, Alfred M
  Drugs: an annotated bibliography and guide to the literature.

  1. Drugs--Bibliography.  2. Drugs--Abstracts.
I. The Sanctuary.  II. Title.
RM300.A47           615'.78      72-13943
ISBN 0-8161-1044-1

*This publication is printed on permanent/durable acid-free paper.*

Copyright © 1973 by The Sanctuary and Alfred M. Ajami

ISBN 0-8161-1044-1

# TABLE of CONTENTS

Note: Numbers appearing in the upper right-hand corner of each card indicate Chapter, Section and entry designations. Example: (II:2) 31 refers to Chapter II, Section 2, entry number 31.

|  | Entry Numbers | Page |
|---|---|---|
| Preface | | v |
| Introduction | | xi |
| Index of Journals and Periodicals Including Abbreviations | | xix |
| **I. Drugs in Physiological Psychology** | | |
| Section 1. Biology and Biochemistry of the Nervous System | 1-25 | 1 |
| Section 2. The Basis of Perception, Sensation, and Memory | 26-42 | 8 |
| Section 3. Drugs and Behavior | 43-82 | 13 |
| **II. Pharmacology: The Study of Drugs** | | |
| Section 1. Alcohol, Nicotine, Caffeine | 83-101 | 25 |
| Section 2. Stimulants | | |
| a) Amphetamines | 102-116 | 30 |
| b) Cocaine | 117-122 | 35 |
| Section 3. Tranquilizers | 123-148 | 37 |
| Section 4. Narcotics | 149-178 | 45 |
| Section 5. Psychedelics | | |
| a) L.S.D. and Related Drugs | 179-204 | 53 |
| b) Mescaline, Mushrooms and Molds | 205-225 | 61 |
| c) Biochemical and Clinical Research with Psychedelics | 226-264 | 67 |

| | | |
|---|---|---|
| Section 6. Marihuana | | |
|   a) Social and Legal Aspects of Marihuana | 265-290 | 80 |
|   b) Biochemical and Clinical Research on Marihuana | 291-303 | 88 |
| Section 7. Inhalants | 304-312 | 93 |
| Section 8. Chemical Identification and Clinical Diagnosis of Psychoactive Drugs | 313-330 | 96 |

III. Drugs in Society
    Section 1. Drugs and the Young    331-368    101
    Section 2. Drugs in the Sociology and Politics of the Counterculture    369-426    112

IV. Cultural and Philosophic Overviews: The Drug Experience    427-529    129

Appendices
    I. Summary of Scientific Information about Drugs    161
    II. Guide to Bibliographic and Search Services    177

Indexes
    Subject Index    181
    Author Index    193

# Preface

In the fall of 1970 Fotis Kafatos, professor of biology at Harvard asked me to lead a seminar in an exciting course offered for only the second time as part of the University's general education program. Natural Sciences 26 was to be a new kind of biology course that would transcend the laboratory and project itself upon a broader arena of human concern. Those of us participating as teachers were called upon to use our analytic skills as scientists to examine a variety of issues on the borderline between the natural and the social sciences. I focused my attention on drugs and the drug culture.

In retrospect, though, the focusing process demanded a special effort to achieve the goals outlined in the course prospectus. "This section of Natural Science 26," I wrote.

> will attempt to reach an understanding of the causes and consequences of perhaps the most talked about public syndrome of the decade - what Timothy Leary called the Turn On, the flash of light, the sudden bolt of chemical ecstasy - psychedelia. The approach to a topic such as this perforce must be

# PREFACE

  interdisciplinary, with almost equal influence placed upon its neurological, pharmacological, historical, social, and political implications.

No doubt it was a large order to fill.

  I began my preparations for the course by visiting the Countway Library at the Harvard Medical School in Boston. After a few hours of intense browsing in the reference room I was impressed by the staggering wealth of information on every conceivable drug related topic available to the public at large through computerized abstracting services. The Excerpta Medica Foundation, the Chemical, Biological and Psychological Abstracts, and the National Library of Medicine literature services are notable among these, for the depth with which they cover monthly more than 5,000 journals, published throughout the world, bearing articles pertinent to the study of drugs. To be sure, I found no shortage of definitive bibliographies. But after suffering considerable eyeball strain while pouring over them in search for a representative sampling of literature references; and after several equally frustrating weeks of chasing down those references in Boston, New York, and Washington libraries; I concluded that the existing bibliographic resources about drugs served no useful purpose to the initiate, regardless of his training. I would have profited more from an annotated, directional guide than from all the exhaustive compilations available to me.

  Here the word "directional" must be underscored. It

# PREFACE

was with it in mind that I embarked upon this project: to compile a short yet comprehensive core bibliography intended to help channel the intellectual needs and interest of a variety of potential readers through the vast morass of scientific, sociological, and cultural studies about drugs. Naturally the particular channeling process under consideration would suffer from unavoidable limitations imposed by my personal biases - the biases of a biologist.. The approach towards compiling this literature guide and the interpretation of the subject matter in the annotations cannot be looked upon as products of professional consensus, but rather only as reflections of the views of an individual scientist whose liberal arts education has been sufficient to help him navigate outside of his field of hormone biochemistry.

As a partial guard against shortsightedness, however, my first step involved a thorough scanning of the literature citation indices. These not only listed the names of authors whose work on pharmacology and on the drug culture is most often quoted, but also the journals in which they have published most frequently. I took care to reflect at least this consensus view in the pages that follow so that the reader can appreciate the more vocal scholars on the subject and learn where their best studies can be found. In this connection it has been encouraging to observe over the past two years that my judgements with regard to author and journal selection for the annotated guide have coincided closely with the judgements of more established scholars.

## PREFACE

The author and journal indices of several monographs about drugs, currently held in high esteem, to my satisfaction are amply reflected in the corresponding indices at the end of this text.

From a qualitative standpoint, on the other hand, the validity of the subject matter and commentary in each of the 529 references included here is more open to challenge. Practically every student in my Natural Sciences 26 seminar and many others in related courses, who have had occasion to use the earlier drafts of this bibliography, has taken issue with one or another of my opinions. Causes for debate, often unknown to myself, appear to be seeded throughout the text. All the better; debate is a powerful tool. One must remember that this is a teaching bibliography, designed with a hope to stimulate thought and discussion. LSD causes genetic damage states a group of scientists in one citation found in Chapter II, while in the next citation the claim is negated by the evidence of another research group. So too an exchange of charges and countercharges characterizes the entries about marihuana, heroin, or the citations of studies on the chemistry of consciousness, the role of drugs in religion, and on other controversial issues. In short, I have attempted to include enough material for individual readers to take adequately documented stands on either side of a critical scientific, social, or philosophic issue pertaining to drugs, regardless of the relationship between their personal biases and my own. Such an opportunity is

## PREFACE

seldom afforded by the massive and in one seating intellectually indigestible bibliographies already on the library stacks.

Once I had satisfied myself that approximately two hundred pages of key references would suffice, the new problem to be resolved in the preparation of this guide became one of organization. Although a number of possibilities for the format of this bibliographic guide are imaginable, I chose the path of least resistance by following closely the format of the general reading list presented to my students in Natural Sciences 26. The course material had been divided into four parts, each of which now constitutes a chapter in this book.

To the extent that this teaching bibliography of the literature on drugs resulted from the collective effort of many people around me, I am not only pleased with it but proud. Acknowledgements are due to the Sanctuary - a youth counseling and education research center in Harvard Square, Cambridge - for sponsoring and promoting this book. I am particularly in debt to the editors of its final stages - Fletcher McLellan and Mary Jane McKinven - who expertly whipped a sloppy and sluggish manuscript into respectability with enthusiasm and record speed.

I wish to thank Professors Lynn M. Riddiford and Carroll M. Williams, whose lectures in human physiology several years ago attracted interest toward the intricacies of the nervous system, and Professor E. J. Corey, who drew my attention to

## PREFACE

the subtleties of organic chemistry. My gratitude also to Professor Richard Schultes, whose work on ethnopharmacology has provided me with constant stimulus, and to Drs. Peter Cherbas, Dennis Crouse, James Hunsley, and Joe Richmond for numerous illuminating discussions. Last but never least, my deep appreciation to friends, many of them from the Sanctuary and from my seminar on drugs - Jeff Blum, Liz Coe, Abigail English, Joan Griffin, Ted Jones, Stephen Langstaff, Martha McCahill, Holly McLellan, Molly Pauker, and especially Peggy Rizza - all of whom more than once came to my rescue.

Alfred M. Ajami, Jr.

September 1972
Cambridge, Massachusetts

# Introduction

Chapter I addresses itself to questions of neurophysiology and neuropharmacology. It is intended in Section 1 to provide an understanding of the nervous system's circuitry and chemistry insofar as they are understood at present. Section 2 illustrates current scientific views of the process by which the circuits and chemical messages are integrated within the brain to produce such complex functions as consciousness, perception, thought, and memory. At the same time the process is described by which these functions can be derailed through specific chemical interactions with particular drug molecules. While Sections 1 and 2 deal with the covert phenomena of the nervous system, neural phenomena not noticeable to the naked eye, Section 3 presents information about several overt phenomena which are the direct results of brain chemistry and which are known collectively as behavior. Of course the process of brain chemistry like any other biological process is not foolproof, and when set awry by genetic or environmental factors, or by drugs, then behavior changes accordingly. Section 3 also examines schizophrenia, psychosis, and drug addiction as examples of aberrant behavior caused by subtle and not yet fully understood changes in the nervous system.

## INTRODUCTION

Chapter II is devoted to pharmacology. The references cited in it were selected with the hope of maximizing an appreciation for such topics as the physical properties; modes of action; medical, non-medical, and ethnic uses; and the dangers of the drugs most frequently consumed throughout the world today: alcohol, nicotine, caffeine, stimulants, amphetamines and cocaine, tranquilizers, narcotics, psychedelics, marihuana, and inhalants. These categories comprise the subject matter of Sections 1 through 7. Section 8 is concerned with a highly technical appraisal of the laboratory and clinical diagnostic procedures available for detecting the abuse of these chemicals.

Throughout Chapter II, I have attempted to convey a feeling for the difficulties encountered by the many researchers and clinicians whose work has been cited. And for the benefit of the reader, at this point I should state that in my opinion the most staggering obstacle to progress in the study of drugs is a conceptual one. The nature of the effects of drugs upon the human organism is so complex that the easy generalizations or simplifications which often emerge even in scientific studies cannot be justified. The cases in which a clearcut answer can be given to the ubiquitous question "How does a drug work?" are few and far between because the overall visible effects of drugs upon their users result from multiple interactions of at least three levels within the body. Each kind of drug can interfere with the normal function of the nervous system; alter the workings of organs like

## INTRODUCTION

individual users. Yet, at least along rough lines, the motivations most often identified by sociologists, psychologists, and psychiatrists fall into two temporal categories. Some are dated; others are timeless. Chapter III embraces the former. I have chosen a representative assortment of references that account for the increase of drug use - whether among students or other segments of the population, whether with legal or illegal drugs - as a rebellious response to the particular pressures and polarizing conflicts and to the sense of personal meaninglessness so often encountered in contemporary society.

To a lesser extent in the same chapter, I have also included suggestive references which examine the phenomenon of drug abuse within the predictable socio-political climate of the future. In the novel entitled Psychedelic-40, for example, drug abuse is depicted as an expression of social conformity, even submission. On a more realistic note in Heyman's essay, "Methadone Maintenance as Law and Order", again the phenomenon of drug abuse carries an equally dangerous right-wing connotation. In particular, the author notes that substitution of methadone for heroin, at the instigation of powerful public and private lobby groups, may be used in the near future as a method of tranquilizing the potentially rebellious ghetto and poor white populations; and a similar sentiment is expressed in the far-reaching study by the Hudson Institute which asserts that twenty or thirty years from now drugs will be used to establish

## INTRODUCTION

and preserve social equilibrium rather than to disrupt it.
Human motivations evolve in response to changes within
the political fabric of society.

But, intuitively, there exist motivations for drug use
which rest free from the restrictions of political eventualities. Those motivations are timeless and intangible.
"The soul of man returns to where it was a child," said
Plato, the Greek philosopher, in describing the results
of excessive drinking of wine. And he continued,

> no experiment is less costly and none shall
> bear fruit more surely and more quickly - if
> we wish to test the different characters of
> men and to judge them and to be guided in the
> art of making them better - than to know them
> in the truth of the drunk.

Chapter IV is dedicated to that ambitious end, providing
the more general phrase "to know them in the truth of the
drug experience" is substituted for the last few words of
Plato's observation. Although the chapter is not organized
into discrete sections, I have included references that
attempt to explain the positive influence of the drug
experience upon man's capacity for artistic creation and
ecstasy. There are also references addressed to the
role of drugs in religion, mysticism, sexuality, and
witchcraft. Certainly for me, the references in this
chapter have been the most rewarding. Through them, more
so than through any of the others, I have been able to
enjoy a fleeting glimpse of the "Turn On" which for
poets, high priests, mystics, madmen, and hippies has

INTRODUCTION

been a daily occurrence.

But on a higher intellectual plane this chapter proves itself worthy of consideration because the material in it as a whole presents a provocative counterargument to one of the central themes in Western culture. Again, Plato described it in a metaphor likening the human soul to a pair of winged horses and a charioteer. One horse "noble and of noble breed" leads upward toward clarity and light. The other, "ignoble and of ignoble origin", leads downward away from clarity toward confusion. And the charioteer struggles to move his chariot in one of the two directions. The prevalent cultural assumption has been that those qualities which make man a unique creature - his capacity for aesthetic creation, for vision, for religious and philosophical activity - have arisen from his desire as the metaphorical charioteer to steer in the direction of the Noble and the Good.

But the phenomenon of the drug experience with all of its ramifications indicates that at least under limited circumstances those admirable capacities find fulfillment also whenever the human soul is drawn by the ignoble horse toward a darker world shrouded with hallucinatory ritual or tainted by madness and depravity. "I know that gold made with fire instead of by the sun is not genuine," said a disciple in a scenario from Thomas Mann's novel Doktor Faustus which is particularly apropos in this context. Mephistopheles replied:

## INTRODUCTION

> Who says so? Has the sun better fire than the kitchen?...Like an innocent do you believe in anything that has nothing to do with hell? Not so! The artist is the brother of the criminal and the madman. Do you presume that any important work was ever wrought except its maker learned to understand the way of the criminal and madman? Morbid and healthy! Without the morbid would life its whole life never have survived.

For those who choose to accept it, there lies the most profound insight to be gained ultimately from a study of the drug culture. The daemon is often as necessary as the angel.

And finally, to conclude this synopsis, I must add that the annotated text of the four chapters just described is complemented by two appendices and three indices. Appendix I offers a summary of the scientific information about drugs treated in Chapter II. Appendix II offers a survey of the drug-oriented bibliographic and abstracting services available at most major public and private libraries. The author index cites over a thousand names, including those of the fifty most prominent and esteemed scholars in the field. The journal index provides familiarity with both technical and non-technical periodicals which regularly publish articles about drugs and the drug culture. And lastly the subject index - tried and tested successfully for two years by frequent visitors to my laboratory - is extensive enough to redeem the text wherever it suffers from lack of organization.

# INDEX OF JOURNALS AND PERIODICALS

Note: Underlining corresponds to abbreviations used in the text.
Numbers refer to entries, not pages.
*Starred journals are those with at least 10% of each issue devoted to articles on subjects about drugs.

Acta Physiologica et Pharmacologica Neerlandica. 244

American Family Physician. 332

Adolescence. 361, 503

American Journal of Clinical Hypnosis. 452

American Journal of Clinical Pathology. 316

American Journal of Nursing. 58

American Journal of Orthopsychiatry. 337, 385

American Journal of Pharmacology. 198

American Journal of Psychiatry. 184, 206, 247, 251, 253, 267, 332, 352, 353, 362, 377

American Journal of Public Health. 349, 350, 365

American Scientist. 36

Angewandte Chemie International Edition in English. 24, 148

Annals of Internal Medicine. 305

Annals of the New York Academy of Science. 229, 235

Archives of Environmental Health. 312

*Archives of General Psychiatry. 52, 87, 156, 171, 195, 255, 291, 300, 344, 358, 363, 368

## INDEX OF JOURNALS AND PERIODICALS

Archives of Neurology and Psychiatry. 85, 488

Arts Magazine. 511

Biochemical Journal. 233

Biochemical Pharmacology. 122

Biological Psychiatry. 32

Boston Globe, Sunday Magazine. 517

Brain. 6

Brain Research. 96, 101

*British Journal of Addictions. 86, 91, 118, 331, 336, 496

British Journal Medical Psychology. 308, 309

*British Journal of Pharmacology. 1, 145

British Journal of Psychiatry. 79

British Medical Bulletin. 249

British Medical Journal. 99

*Bulletin on Narcotics. 120, 159, 208, 323, 515, 516

Canadian Medical Association Journal. 119, 127, 128

Canadian Journal of Behavioral Science. 351

Children. 345

Clinical Chemistry. 49

*Clinical Pharmacology and Therapeutics. 13, 117, 130, 132

Comparative Biochemistry and Physiology. 21

Comparative Psychiat. 183, 245

Crime and Delinquency. 333, 424

Current Anthropology. 211

Diseases of the Nervous System. 30, 294

Economic Botany. 478

Esquire. 384

## INDEX OF JOURNALS AND PERIODICALS

ETC. 490

Existential Psychiatry. 464, 510

Experientia. 227

Experimental Medicine and Surgery. 31, 42, 242

Farmakologiya i Toksikologiya. (USSR). 295

Federation Proceedings. 14, 167

Harvard Review. 401

Health Education Journal. 372

Human Biology. 121

International Journal of Addictions. 126, 310, 347, 357

International Review of Neurobiology. 115, 257

International Journal of Neuropsychiatry. 475

International Journal of Parapsychology. 179, 185

Journal of Abnormal Psychology. 182

Journal of the American College Health Association. 279, 283, 355, 358

Journal of the American Chemical Society. 146

Journal of the American Medical Association. 45, 54, 152, 153, 162, 174, 328, 346, 397, 398, 454

Journal of Chromatographic Science. 322

Journal of Clinical and Experimental Psychiatry. 193

Journal of Comparative and Physiological Psychiatry. 131, 147

Journal of Consultational and Clinical Psychiatry. 348

Journal of Forensic Medicine. 324, 325

*Journal of Forensic Science. 314, 318, 320, 329, 330, 455

*Journal of Health and Social Behavior. 177, 338, 489

Journal of Medical Times. 317

Journal of Mental Science. 261

## INDEX OF JOURNALS AND PERIODICALS

*Journal of Nervous and Mental Disease  213, 252

Journal of Neuropsychiatry.  472

Journal of New Drugs.  387

Journal of Obstretrics and Gynaecology of the British Commonwealth.  165

Journal of Occupational Medicine.  326

*Journal of Pharmaceutical Sciences.  188, 208, 303, 321

*Journal of Pharmacology and Experimental Therapeutics.  143, 155

Journal of Philosophy.  512

*Journal of Psychedelic Drugs.  107, 113

Journal of Psychology.  197

Journal of Psychosomatic Medicine.  151

Journal of Social Issues.  412, 421, 495

Life Sciences.  135

Look.  364

Journal of Consultational and Clinical Psychiatry.  348

Medicina et Pharmacologia Experimentalis.  108

Mental Hygiene.  158

*Nature.  3, 23, 37, 48, 51, 102, 110-112, 136, 138, 142, 237, 238, 248, 256, 262, 281, 289, 297, 343

Neuropsychologia.  254

Neuroscience Research Program Bulletin.  5

New England Journal of Medicine.  65, 172

New York Times.  469

Pediatrics.  311

*Pharmacological Reviews.  116, 124, 127, 139, 140, 161, 217, 240

Physiological Reviews.  33

## INDEX OF JOURNALS AND PERIODICALS

Playboy. 409, 519

Proceedings of the National Academy of Science. 232, 259, 260

Proceedings of the Society for Experimental Biology and Medicine. 264

Progress in Brain Research. 3

*Psychedelic Review. 214, 215, 223, 373, 414, 428, 479, 484, 494, 498, 505, 506

Psychiatric Quarterly. 35, 466

Psychiatry. 222

Psychoanalysis and Psychoanalytic Reviews. 313

Psychoanalytic Reviews. 370

Psychological Medicine. 76

*Psychopharmacologia. 104, 105, 209, 250, 258

*Psychopharmacology Bulletin. 70

Psychosomatic Medicine. 59

*Quarterly Journal of Studies on Alcohol. 85, 93, 94, 134, 144, 269

Reporter. 386

Review of Existential Psychology and Psychiatry. 168, 453, 480, 518

Rolling Stone Magazine. 382

Saturday Evening Post. 196

*Science. 8, 19, 34, 38, 44, 47, 67, 72, 98, 114, 175, 207, 218, 219, 226, 228, 230, 234, 236, 239, 241, 243, 263, 275, 293, 296, 298, 299, 304, 315, 399, 403, 422, 457

Seminars in Psychiatry. 173

Scientific American. 9, 18, 28, 123, 133, 166, 176, 273, 432

Social Problems. 292

Society. 390, 429

## INDEX OF JOURNALS AND PERIODICALS

Sociological and Social Research. 282, 306

Sociological Quarterly. 487, 525

Southern Medical Journal. 141

Sports Illustrated. 340

Texas Medicine. 319, 335

Zeitschrift fur Naturforschung. 231

# CHAPTER I

# Drugs in Physiological Psychology

Section 1: Biology and Biochemistry
of the Nervous System

(I:1)1

Adam, H. M., and H. K. A. Hye. 1966. Concentration of histamine in different parts of the brain and hypophysis of the cat and its modification by drugs. Brit. J. Pharmacol. 18:137-152.

The product of histamine, a neurotransmitter, is sensitive to various drugs. The authors demonstrate how the tranquilizer reserpine causes histamine depletion in certain important regions of the brain while another tranquilizer, chlorpromazine (thorazine) increases the amine's concentration in the same regions.

(I:1)2

Axelrod, J. 1964. The uptake and release of catecholamines and the effects of drugs. Prog. Brain. Res. 8:81-89.

A short, general review of the chemical communication between nerve cells.

(I:1)3

Baker, R. W., C. H. Chothia, P. Pauling, and T. J. Petcher. 1971. Structure and activity of muscarinic stimulants. Nature 230:439-445.

The junction between the parasympathetic nerves and the autonomic (involuntary) nervous system and the autonomic organs is known as the muscarinic junction, because the natural substance muscarine from the mushroom amanita muscaria stimulates the release of acetylcholine, the principal neurotransmitter of the central nervous system, across that junction. The article reviews current information pertaining to that stimulating effect (43 references).

(I:1)4

Black, P., ed. 1969. Drugs and the brain. The Johns Hopkins Press, Baltimore.

An up-to-date edition of the principal scientific studies of the many interactions between depressant, stimulant or psychedelic drugs and the normal biochemical functions of the brain; also a sourcebook and bibliographic guide.

(I:1)5

Bloom, F. E., L. L. Iversen, and F. O. Schmitt, eds. 1970. Macromolecules in synaptic transmission. Neurosci. Res. Prog. Bull. 8(1).

A definitive, 130 page treatment. This volume reviews how nerve impulses are transmitted from one nerve cell to another at the synapse. The bibliography includes pertinent references up to September, 1970.

(I:1)6

Bradley, P. B., and J. Elkes. 1957. The effect of some drugs on the electrical activity of the brain. Brain 80:77-117.

This article is a detailed compendium of neurophysical data. Patterns of electrical activity generated by various drugs, the psychedelics in particular, are compared and contrasted to the normal electrical rhythms of wakefulness and sleep in cats and monkeys.

(I:1)7

Clark, W. G. and J. del Giudice. 1970. Principles of psychopharmacology. Academic Press, New York.

Subtitled "a textbook for physicians, medical students, and behavioral scientists," this is the most comprehensive collective volume currently available, a fact reflected both in the organization of the text and in the thoroughness of the appendices. Forty pages of references to key reviews, monographs, and texts in the scientific and non-scientific literature on drugs. Additional appendices report on annuals and serials, core journals and bibliographic and literature research aids.

(I:1)8

De Robertis, E. 1971. Molecular biology of synaptic receptors. Science 171:963-971.

> The physical and chemical properties of synaptic receptors are described, insofar as they are currently understood. A highly specialized article, it also includes a critique of the scientific literature and 54 citations to research on the subject over the last ten years.

(I:1)9

Eccles, J. 1964. The synapse. Sci. Am. 212: 56-70.

> The mechanism by which one nerve cell transmits impulses to another is examined with respect to the junction between the two cells. Technical, but readable. Eccles is a recognized authority.

(I:1)10

Folch, Pi. J., ed. 1961. The chemical pathology of the nervous system. Pergamon Press, New York.

> This textbook amply documents the biochemical bases for abnormal behavior. Although out of date, it provides background information useful in understanding how this field of study has been evolving over the last decade.

(I:1)11

Galambos, R. 1962. Nerves and muscles. Anchor-Doubleday, Garden City, New York.

> This text is often used as supplementary reading in introductory courses on the physiological basis of psychology. It describes best the neural integrating mechanisms that control muscle function.

(I:1)12

Gardner, E. 1963. Fundamentals of neurology. Saunders, Philadelphia.

Another introductory text to the subject. Its index and bibliography are recommended as a guide to the classical literature on neurology.

(I:1)13

Goldstein, L., H. B. Murphree, H. A. Sugarman, C C. Pfeiffer, and E. H. Jenney. 1963. Quantitative electroencephalographic analysis of naturally occurring (schizophrenic) and drug-induced psychotic states in human males. Clin. Pharmacol. Therapeut. 4:10-21.

The assertion that drug-induced and naturally occurring psychotic states share a physiological basis is tested and partially confirmed by this study.

(I:1)14

Green, J. P. 1964. Histamine and the nervous system. Fed. Proc. 23:1095-1102.

Data linking histamine--an endogenous amine in body chemistry--with the functioning of the nervous system. Also a discussion of drugs including amphetamines and LSD.

(I:1)15

Green, J. P. 1970. in A. Lajtha, ed. Handbook of neurochemistry. Plenum Press, New York. Vol. IV:221-224.

A more extensive and explicit treatment of subjects introduced in #14 above. Note the section describing the involvement of histamine in schizophrenia and similar, artificially-induced psychic states.

(I:1)16

Guyton, A. C. 1969. Function of the human body. Saunders, Philadelphia.

> A simplified text on human physiology. Chapter 6, The Nervous System, clearly presents a detailed review of the subject in a manner especially suited for readers with little scientific background.

(I:1)17

Himwich, H. E. and W. A. Himwich, eds. 1964. Biogenic amines. Elsevier Publishing Company, Amsterdam.

> A classic text on the functions of the body's own amines--dopamine, norepinephrine, acetylcholine, serotonin--in normal physiological and psychological processes (A collection of papers).

(I:1)18

Luria, A. R. 1970. The functional organization of the brain. Sci. Am. 3:66-78.

> The sensory and motor functions of the human brain are well localized, but the site of more complex functions such as speech and writing remain obscure. Investigations of injuries to the brain provide clues to how such systems are organized. The article serves as a quick guide to the gross anatomy of the higher centers controlling body functions.

(I:1)19

Pauling, L. 1968. Orthomolecular psychiatry. Varying the concentrations of substances normally present in the human body may control mental diseases. Science 160:265-271.

> A seminal thinker in the study of molecular relationships, Nobel laureate Linus Pauling proposes the view that sanity depends upon a delicate balance between concentrations of certain compounds of great importance to the body (biogenic amines). Perhaps leaves the unfortunate impression that the psyche is merely a function of body chemistry.

(I:1)20

Penfield, W., and L. Roberts. 1959. Speech and brain mechanisms. Princeton University Press, Princeton.

Dr. Penfield and his collaborator discuss the functional mapping of the human cortex. Their studies of hundreds of patients during the course of open brain surgery have yielded a correlation between specific regions of the brain and certain conscious activities like speech, hearing, and muscle movements. The book represents one of the most exciting experimental approaches in physiological psychology.

(I:1)21

Pscheidt, G. R. 1960. Comparative aspects of selected psychoactive compounds: biogenic amines, monoamine oxidase inhibitors, and LSD. Comp. Biochem. Physiol. 24:249-265.

Reviews the biochemical and physiological investigations of disruption of normal integration of nervous system functions in represenative species of each phylum of the animal kingdom. There is an extensive bibliography.

(I:1)22

Purpura, D. P. 1965. Electrophysiological analysis of psychotogenic drug action. Arch. Neurol. Psychiat. 75:122-131.

Purpura reports his study of the effect of LSD on the visual and auditory systems of the cat. Low doses of the psychedelic facilitated electrophysiological responses to light and sound, while high doses enhanced responses to photic stimuli and depressed responses to sound.

(I:1)23

Rang, H. P. 1971. Drug receptors and their function. Nature 231:91-96.

    There have been various theories about the way in which drugs exert their effects. The currently accepted theory calls for drugs to act as competitors for the receptor sites in the nervous system that are normally only available to the body's own neurotransmitters. If recent progress in the isolation and characterization of receptors continues, it should soon be possible to look directly at the interaction between drugs and tissues.

(I:1)24

Seiler, N., L. Denusch, and H. Schneider. 1971. Biochemistry and function of biogenic amines in the central nervous system. Angew. Chem. Int. Ed. Eng. 10:51-66.

    Another review of information on the chemical mechanisms by which sensory information is transmitted within the nervous system. Its chief merit is the presentation of vast amounts of information by way of readable charts and tables. 264 references are cited.

(I:1)25

Smythies, J. R., ed. 1970. The mode of action of psychotomimetic drugs. Neurosci. Res. Prog. Bull. 8(2).

    This is an indispensable paperback both in its scope and content. It was based on a symposium in which practically all of the recognized authorities in the field participated. The topics covered include drug electrophysiology, biochemistry, structure-activity relationships, metabolism, and qualitative effects. A lengthy bibliography is included at the end of the text.

Section 2:  The Basis of Perception,
           Sensation, and Memory

(I:2)26

Adrian, E. D. 1949. The basis of sensation.
    The action of the sense organs. Christophers, London.

    Considered a classic in the field of
    perception physiology, Adrian's work is
    noted for its treatment of pain and "painful" psychic states.

(I:2)27

Chow, K. L., and A. L. Leinman, eds. 1970.
    The structural and functional organization
    of the neocortex. Neurosci. Res. Prog. Bull.
    8(3).

    A short, comprehensive review of the information currently available about vision and
    hearing. Several sections of the book are
    devoted to morphology and circuitry of the
    nervous system. Others discuss how the inputs from the eyes and ears are interpreted
    within the brain of higher animals. A detailed bibliography on the pertinent scientific literature is included.

(I:2)28

Eccles, J. 1958. The physiology of imagination.
    Sci. Am. 199(3):135-146.

    Electrical waves, traveling on multilane pathways among the 10 billion cells
    of the brain cortex, correspond to the
    "experience of mind." An excellent introduction; some biological data given is now
    outdated.

(I:2)29

Eccles, J., ed. 1966. Brain and conscious experience. Springer-Verlag, New York.

    Twenty-one lectures followed by transcripts of group discussions on each. Lucid prose and comprehensive information. An outstanding summary of research on the subjective organization of the brain.

(I:2)30

Fischer, R. 1969. The perception-hallucination continuum, a re-examination. Dis. Nerv. Syst. 30:161-171.

    In this review article, the old concept of hallucinations as "perceptions" without an object is revised in favor or the operational definition, "sensations without action." Thus the sensation/activity ratio gradually increases on the continuum and is highest during hallucinatory experiences and any method or mechanism that increases the ratio can elicit hallucinations.

(I:2)31

Gotthelf, T. 1969. The continuity of fantasy: dreams and dreaming in the arts. Exp. Med. Surg. 27:3-12.

    The relationship between dreams, natural and drug-induced, and the creative process. A convenient summary of theories presented less succintly in various articles and monographs.

(I:2)32

Itil, T. M. 1969. Digital computer "sleep prints" and psychopharmacology. Biol. Psychiat. 1:91-95.

    Describes the quantification of subjective responses to psychoactive drugs during sleep. Each type of drug elicits a particular set of biochemical impulses within the brain which can be recorded and preserved as the "fingerprints" of ideas.

(I:2)33

Jouvet, M. 1967. Neurophysiology of the states of sleep. Physiol. Revs. 47:117-777.

    A lengthy documentary of brain activity during sleep and an equally impressive bibliography, by one of the more competent authorities on the subject.

(I:2)34

Jouvet, M 1969. Biogenic amines and the states of sleep. Science 163:32-41.

    In a distillation of his longer review (#33 above), Jouvet reports on pharmacological and neurophysiological studies which suggest a relationship between brain serotonin and sleep. The effects of drugs on the brain's serotonin concentration are also discussed.

(I:2)35

Kass, W. 1970. Interrelationship of hallucinations and dreams in spontaneously hallucinating patients. Psychiat. Quart. (Suppl.) 44:488-499.

    The article provides background information and supporting evidence to the topic described in the title.

(I:2)36

McGeer, P. L. 1971. The chemistry of mind. Amer. Scientist 59:221-229.

    A simplified account of how modifying the activity of supposed chemical transmitter agents can alter mood and motor activity. This article may also serve as an easy review of basic neurophysiology.

(I:2) 37

Oswald, I. 1969. Human brain protein, drugs and dreams. Nature 223:893-897.

Recovery of normal sleep after drugs takes many weeks. The author cites evidence toward this conclusion in a discussion of the effects of amphetamines (dexedrine), anti-depressants (imipramine), hypnotics (nitrazepan), and sedatives (barbiturates), advancing the claim that these compounds may hinder brain-protein synthesis, with the result that "the healing of hurt minds proceeds by processes equally as slow" as the healing of hurt brain cells.

(I:2) 38

Schildkraut, J. J., and S. S. Kety. 1967. Biogenic amines and emotion. Science 156:21-30.

A detailed review article discussing the relationship between biogenic amines of the brain and the affective (behavioral) state. The function of tranquilizers and stimulants is discussed with reference to clinical studies on representative patients with affective disorders. A bibliography of 141 titles.

(I:2) 39

Schmitt, F. O. ed. 1967. Macromolecular specificity and biological memory. The MIT Press. Cambridge, Mass.

Although a decade out of date, this volume will serve as a valuable introduction to both the research and the researchers in neurochemistry and neurophysiology. The principle merit of this 120 page publication lies in the lucidity with which the various contributions present the molecular basis of such processes as biological coding, thought and memory.

(I:2) 40

Simon, A., C. C. Herbert, and R. Straus, eds. 1961. The physiology of emotion. Charles C. Thomas, Springfield, Illinois.

    An anthology carefully describing the causes--natural or drug-induced--of various emotional states. One of the better standard reference works.

(I:2) 41

Tart, C. T., ed. 1969. Altered states of consciousness: a book of readings. Wiley and Son, New York.

    A collection of essays on dreams, meditation, hypnosis, and psychedelics. Articles by Tart himself appear on the following topics: "Psychedelic Experiences Associated with a Novel Hypnotic Procedure, Mutual Hypnosis"; "The Effects of Marihuana on Consciousness"; and "The 'High Dreams': a New State of Consciousness." An outstanding and up-to-date bibliography.

(I:2) 42

Whitman, R. M., M. Kramer, P. H. Ornstein, and B. J. Baldridge. 1969. Drugs and dream content. Exp. Med. Surg. 27: 210-223.

    Observations on the ability of the mind to have an endopsychic perception of itself under the influence of LSD, opium, stimulants and other drugs.

Section 3: Drugs and Behavior

(I:3) 43

Ausubel, D. P. 1958. Drug addiction. Random House, New York.

The factual material is much outdated, but a succinct, sensitive treatment makes this worth reading.

(I:3) 44

Beecher, H. K. 1952. Experimental pharmacology and measurement of the subjective response. Science 116:157-162.

On pain and pleasure. May be considered a summary of Beecher's 1959 book (see #46 below).

(I:3) 45

Beecher, H. K. 1955. Appraisal of drugs intended to alter subjective responses, symptoms. J. Amer. Med. Ass. 158:399-401.

Together with #44 above, sums up the known clinical material on pain and its close counterpart, pleasure.

(I:3) 46

Beecher, H. K. 1959. Measurement of subjective responses. Oxford University Press, London.

> Still the best book of its kind, though much updated by recent research. Beecher has succeeded in describing the phenomenology of pleasure and pain, and gives valuable insights into the modification of these subjective states by analgesic, stimulating and psychotomimetic drugs. See especially his chapters on the "pain experience." A massive bibliography of 1,063 references dating from 1800.

(I:3) 47

Beecher, H. K. 1969. Human studies. Science 164:1256-1258.

> Although not directly addressed to the issue of research with psychoactive drugs, this article does cover all the important ethical questions raised by experimentation with behavioral drugs on human beings. Dr. Beecher argues that clear legislation is necessary for the protection of both the investigator and his subject.

(I:3) 48

Boueton, A. A. 1971. Biochemical research in schizophrenia. Nature 231:22-23.

> Schizophrenia is still a loosely defined and little understood group on mental diseases, but a great deal of information is accumulating about the biochemical abnormalities which might be characteristic of so-called schizophrenics. The most conspicuous of these "abnormalities," examined in this article, is the appearance of amines in the urine of schizophrenics, which are structurally related to known psychoactive materials. 191 references are cited.

(I:3) 49

Bryson, G. 1972. Biogenic amines in normal
and abnormal behavioral states. Clin.
Chem. 17:5-26.

The author appraises the involvement of
the biogenic amines--acetylcholine,
epinephrine, norepinephrine, dopamine,
serotonin, and gamma-aminobutyric acid--
in behavioral states. Also, aberrant
catecholamine metabolism and structural
differences in related psychotomimetic
substances are considered with particular
regard to schizophrenia and depression.
The principal advantage of this review
over others is its 258 article bibliography.

(I:3) 50

Byrd, O. E. 1970. Medical readings on drug
abuse. Addison-Wesley, Reading, Massachusetts.

A detailed collection of abstracts of
medical and scientific journal articles
on the adverse effects of all categories
of drugs. Non-subjective, and the material is presented without comment. Of
bibliographic interest.

(I:3) 51

Collier, H. O. J. 1968. Supersensitivity
and dependence. Nature 220:228-231.

The article presents a physiological
definition of addiction as a function
of the interaction of a drug with the
normal flow of neurotransmitter substances. Dr. Collier advances the
possibility, with the aid of several
plausible models, that the psychic
effects of a drug arise in a way com-
parable to its physical effects. Addiction is thus construed as a function of chemical supersensitivity rather
than of sociological or psychic malad-
justment.

(I:3) 52

Coppen, A., A. J. Prange, P. C. Whybrow, and
    R. Noguera. 1972. Abnormalities of
    indoleamines in affective disorders.
    Arch. Gen. Psychiat. 26:474-478.

    A highly technical article which explores the extent to which abnormalities in the body's ability to metabolize serotonin are related to affective disorders, mania, and depression. This study also is recommended because it offers a bibliographic distillation of 43 recent publications concerning the topic under consideration.

(I:3) 53

Cutting, W. C. 1967. Handbook of pharmacology. 3rd ed. Appleton-Century-Crofts, New York.

    A survey of the pharmacological actions of drugs. Not an in-depth study, but easy to use, and particularly good for its presentation of structural formulae.

(I:3) 54

Eddy, N. B. 1957. "Addiction producing" versus "habit forming". J. Am. Med. Assoc. 163:1622-1623.

    A brief essay attempting to clarify one of the most troublesome terminological problems in the study of drug abuse.

(I:3) 55

Efron, D. H., ed. 1967. Ethnopharmacologic search for psychoactive drugs. Public Health Serv. Pub. No. 1645. Dept. of Health, Education and Welfare, U.S. Government Printing Office, Washington, D.C.

Few multidisciplinary volumes can boast such a distinguished list of contributors. An essential reference work for any study of the medical, scientific, and sociological aspects of psychoactive drug use. See especially the chapters: "Historical Survey"; "The Botanical Origins of South American Snuffs"; "Nutmeg as a Psychoactive Drug"; and "Fly Agaric and Man".

(I:3) 56

Efron, D. H., ed. 1968. Psychopharmacology. A review of progress. Public Health Serv. Pub. No. 1836. Dept. of Health, Education and Welfare, U.S. Government Printing Office, Washington, D.C.

A massive volume of 1342 pages covering the following topics: neuroanatomical and biochemical pharmacology, drugs and behavior, antineurotic agents, ethical and legal considerations, electroneurological indicators of drug action, toxicology, antidepressant agents, alcohol and addiction, memory and learning, research methodology in human psychopharmacology, antipsychotic agents, and psychotomimetics. Recommended as a portable encyclopedia.

(I:3) 57

Ellis, E. S. 1946. Ancient anodynes. Heinemann, London.

The author cites passages from documents of classical antiquity and their modern commentators attesting to the use of poppy, mandragora, belladona, cannabis, hyoscyamus, datura, mescal, and other drugs since the beginning of recorded history.

(I:3) 58

Fort, J. 1971. Comparison chart of major
    substances used for mind alteration.
    Amer. J. Nursing 71:1740-1741.

    One of the more useful charts
    available to date. The doses and
    effects of the following drug types
    are compared: alcohol, caffeine,
    nicotine, sedatives, stimulants,
    tranquilizers, marihuana, narcotics,
    hallucinogens, antidepressants, and
    inhalants.

(I:3) 59

Glassman, A. 1969. Indoleamines and
    affective disorders. Psychosom.
    Med. 31:107-114.

    The effects of LSD, psilocybin
    and related indoles on emotional
    and behavioral responses discussed
    in a concise review of recent material.
    Valuable for bibliographic purposes.

(I:3) 60

Goodman, L. S., and A. Gilman. 1970.
    The pharmacological basis of thera-
    peutics. 4th ed. MacMillan, New York.

    Presents detailed summaries and
    bibliographies on the effects,
    mode of action, and clinical uses
    of drugs. Superb indexing; highly
    recommended as a general reference
    for initial inquiry. (The 3rd edition
    is also good.)

(I:3) 61

Harris, R. T., W. M. McIsaac, and D. R. Schuster. 1970. Drug dependence. University of Texas Press, Austin.

A multiphasic study treating in depth the biological, behavioral and social aspects of dependence on a wide variety of drugs. The sections on behavior are particularly well-organized and informative.

(I:3) 62

Himwich, H. E., S. S. Kety, and J. R. Smythies, eds. 1967. Biogenic amines and schizophrenia. Pergamon Press, New York.

A thorough anthology of publications from medical and scientific journals. The editors plausibly relate the chemistry of the brain to the vicissitudes of the schizophrenic personality. A complete bibliography and competent index.

(I:3) 63

Hoffer, A., and H. Osmond. 1960. The chemical basis of clinical psychiatry. Charles C. Thomas, Springfield, Illinois.

Drug therapy as a psychiatric tool. Extensive bibliography.

(I:3) 64

Canadian Government Commission of Inquiry. 1971. The non-medical use of drugs. Interim report. Penguin, New York.

A complete, informative, and up-to-date listing of drugs (including alcohol, barbiturates, marihuana, etc.), their use and abuse, and the sociology which surrounds them.

(I:3)  65

Kety, S. S. 1967. Current biochemical approaches to schizophrenia. New Eng. J. Med. 276:325-331.

A wealth of information condensed into a few pages. The discussion of disturbances in amine metabolism permits several parallels to be drawn between schizophrenia and the symptoms of drug abuse.

(I:3)  66

Laurie, P. 1967. Drugs: medical, psychological and social facts. Penguin Books, Baltimore.

Adequate but difficult reading. As with all such summaries, the tendency is toward oversimplification.

(I:3)  67

Leake, C. D. 1961. The scientific status of pharmacology. Science 134:2069-2080.

Another historical review addressing itself to the men and the circumstances that transformed a branch of alchemy into the modern science of pharmacology. This article is noteworthy because the author looks at pharmacology as a body of specific, applied knowledge developing in step with general scientific discoveries about cellular, tissue, organism, and social levels of living organization.

(I:3)  68

Leride, J., B. C. Schiele, and L. Bouthilet, eds. 1971. Establishing the efficacy of psychotropic agents. U.S. Government Printing Office, Washington, D.C.

An extensive assessment of the methods currently used to evaluate the usefulness and safety of psychoactive chemicals. The chapters on the design of laboratory and chemical experiments is noteworthy.

(I:3) 69

Lewin, L. 1931. Phantastica--narcotic and
stimulating drugs, their use and abuse.
Kegan Paul, French and Turner, London.
(Reprinted 1964 by Kegan Paul and Routledge).

Phantastica first appeared in German in
1924 and sparked today's extensive interdisciplinary interest in narcotics and
hallucinogens. A novel publication, it
presented the total botanical, chemical,
historical and sociological picture on
some 28 plants used internationally for
their intoxicating or stimulating properties.

(I:3) 70

National Institute of Mental Health. 1971.
Pharmacotherapy of children. Psychopharmacol. Bull. 7(2):14-28.

The main focus of this bibliography is
on the drug treatment of hyperactivity
in children. Although studies of the
mentally retarded and studies with
general implications for diagnosis and
treatment are also included.

(I:3) 71

Lingeman, R. R. 1969. Drugs from A to Z:
a dictionary. McGraw-Hill, New York.

An expanded glossary of scientific
information, historical lore and hippie
slang, but not as comprehensive as the
title would suggest; e.g. under "Soma",
"an intoxicating beverage...from an
unknown plant (possibly Asclepias acida
or cannabis)". Lingeman fails to note
Gordon Wasson has already demonstrated
that soma is fly agaric, a concoction
prepared from the mushroom Amanita muscaria, and that "Soma" is the trade name
for a sedative.

(I:3) 72

Modell, W. 1963. Hazards of new drugs.
　　Science 139:1180-1185.

　　The author devotes this powerful article
to the proposition that "no drug, no matter how thoroughly tested by time or
trial, is absolutely safe." In particular,
he cautions over-eager physicians, who
are among the principal promoters of new
drugs, to avoid the lures of pharmaceutical pressure groups and to be careful
of overstating themselves in research
publications on the use of novel therapeutic agents. "If we are to avoid the
dangers and have the fullest possible
benefit of modern medication," he notes,
"we must have the scientist, for only
he can deal safely and effectively with
the output of today's pharmaceutical
chemist." Numerous examples are cited
where harmful drugs that affect behavior
have been used indiscriminately.

(I:3) 73

National Library of Medicine Literature
　　Searches. 1969. Psychotropic drug addiction or withdrawal symptoms in man.
　　U.S. Dep. of Health, Education, and
　　Welfare, Washington, D.C.

　　A bibliography (L.S. No. 3-69) covering
207 references from January 1964 to
August 1968.

(I:3) 74

National Library of Medicine Literature
　　Searches. 1969. Psychotherapy in drug
　　addiction or abuse. U.S. Dep. of Health,
　　Education, and Welfare, Washington, D.C.

　　A bibliography (L.S. No. 2-69) citing
287 references from January 1964 to
August 1968.

(I:3) 75

Root, W. S., and F. G. Hoffmann, eds. 1963. Physiological pharmacology. Academic Press, New York.

> A complete, multi-volume handbook on drugs and their effects, covering most of the material on depressants and stimulants available to the date of publication.

(I:3) 76

Shepherd, M. 1972. The classification of psychotropic drugs. Psychological Med. 2:96-110.

> An historical review of the semantic pitfalls inherent in the existing classification scheme for various kinds of pharmacological agents. The traditional subdivisions are re-examined by the author with an eye towards developing a new classficatory system. The article is followed by a 50-entry bibliography on pharmacological semantics.

(I:3) 77

Solomon, P., ed. 1966. Psychiatric drugs. Grune & Stratton, New York.

> A selection of multidisciplinary, general essays on psychotherapeutics.

(I:3) 78

Steinberg, H., A. V. S de Rench, and J. Knights, eds. 1964. Animal behavior and drug action. Little, Brown and Company, Boston.

> The study of animal behavior can be successfully applied to test the hallucinogenic potential of a new compound for humans. This anthology of papers by prominent investigators describes the battery of tests, mostly on rats, now available for such purposes. A useful and extensive index and bibliography.

(I:3) 79

Smythies, J. R., U. S. Johnston, and R. J.
    Bradley. 1969. Behavioral models of
    psychosis. Brit. J. Psychiat. 115:55-68.

   A handy summary of the symptoms of
   psychoses. Offers several views of
   the professional terminology associated with their description.

(I:3) 80

Uhr, L., and J. G. Miller, eds. 1960.
    Drugs and behavior. Wiley and Sons,
    New York.

   A valuable reference work, particularly
   strong in information about stimulants
   and tranquilizers and their physiological and behavioral effects.

(I:3) 81

Unger, S., A. Kurland, I. Shaffer, C. Savage,
    S. Wolf, R. Leihy, O. McCabe and H. Shock.
    1966. Psychedelic therapy. Third Conference
    on Research in Psychotherapy, Chicago.

   An exhaustive symposium on the current
   state of this approach to changing de-
   viant behavior by the use of drugs.

(I:3) 82

Wolstenholme, G. E., ed. 1958. The neuro-
    logical basis of behavior. J. & A.
    Churchill, London.

   A generally available textbook treatment of an introductory nature, covering
   thoroughly the interaction of drugs and
   behavior. Redeemed by its informative
   index.

# CHAPTER II

# Pharmacology: the Study of Drugs

## DRUGS: AN ANNOTATED BIBLIOGRAPHY AND GUIDE

Section 1: Alcohol, Nicotine, and Caffeine

(II:1) 83

Abramson, H. 1967. The use of LSD in psychotherapy and alcoholism. Bobbs-Merrill, New York.

This volume is considered to be one of the standard reference works on the subject of LSD psychotherapy. Also includes considerable background information on the etiology (i.e., the sequential unfolding of causes and consequences) of various mental diseases as well as alcoholism.

(II:1) 84

Addiction Research Foundation. 1971. Interaction of alcohol and other drugs. Addiction Research Foundation, Toronto.

An annotated bibliography providing 1,050 articles about the problem of alcohol and drug use. It is the third in a series of similar bibliographies.

(II:1) 85

Boyd, J. E. 1970. A multidimensional explication of popular notions of alcoholism. Quart. J. Stud. Alc. 31:876-889.

An extensive study, with detailed references to the literature on the subject over the last twenty years.

(II:1) 86

Burnett, G. B. 1970. The pharmacology of
    disulfiram in the treatment of alco-
    holism. Brit. J. Addict. 65:281-288.

    The drug known by trade name as Anta-
    buse makes alcoholics "allergic" to
    ethanol and therefore can be used as
    an inducement to withdrawal from the
    habit.

---

(II:1) 87

Goodwin, D. 1971. Is alcoholism hereditary?
    Arch. Gen. Psychiat. 25:545-549.

    A review and critique of the influence
    of heredity on alcoholism - a disease
    presumed to be familial since studies
    have repeatedly shown a high prevalence
    of alcoholism among the relatives of
    alcoholics. Thirty-five publications
    are cited.

---

(II:1) 88

Hoffer, A. and H. Osmond. 1968. New hope
    for alcoholics. University Books,
    New York.

    A study of the use and effectiveness
    of psychedelic drugs in the treatment
    of alcoholism. Detailed discussions
    of particular cases and approaches to
    therapy.

---

(II:1) 89

Israel, Y., and J. Mardones, eds. 1971.
    Basic aspects of alcoholism. Wiley-
    Interscience, New York.

    A comprehensive sourcebook on
    alcoholism, written from a multi-
    disciplinary point of view.

(II:1) 90

Jones, K., L. W. Shainberg, and C. O. Byer. 1970. Drugs, alcohol, and tobacco. Canfield Press, San Francisco.

Recommended as a source reference to the use and consequences of the social drugs--alcohol and tobacco-- prior to the advent of pot.

(II:1) 91

Kielholz, P. 1970. Alcohol and depression. Brit. J. Addict. 65:187-193.

A general, comprehensive review of alcohol as a depressant.

(II:1) 92

Lucia, S. 1963. Alcohol and civilization. McGraw-Hill, New York.

A historical monograph, particularly illustrative with regard to the social function of alcohol as an intoxicant.

(II:1) 93

Lundquist, F. 1971. Influence of ethanol on carbohydrate metabolism. Quart. J. Stud. Alc. 32:1-12.

On the biochemistry of how excess alcohol intake leads to undesirable physical conditions such as obesity or liver malfunction.

(II:1) 94

MacLean, J. R., D. C. MacDonald, U. P. Byrne, and A. M. Hubbard. 1961. The use of LSD-25 in the treatment of alcoholism and other psychiatric problems. Quart. J. Stud. Alc. 22: 34-45.

A short survey with a good critical appraisal of the clinical studies conducted throughout the fifties in psychedelic therapy as treatment for alcoholism.

(II:1) 95

National Library of Medicine Literature Searches. 1970. Drug therapy of alcoholism. U.S. Dep. of Health, Education and Welfare, Washington, D.C.

A bibliography (L.S. No. 70-71) citing 323 references from January 1967 to December 1969.

(II:1) 96

Palaic, D. 1971. Effect of ethanol on metabolism and subcellular distribution of serotonin in rat brain. Brain Res. 25:381-366.

Chronic administration of ethanol irreparably disrupts the balance between biosynthesis and metabolism of serotonin. The drug poisons these critical biochemical interactions at the level of the synapse in the brain.

(II:1) 97

Roueche, B. 1960. The neutral spirit: a portrait of alcohol. Little, Brown and Company, New York.

Alcohol may look handsome when contrasted to heroin or other severe addictive drugs, but the author notes in several hundred pages of elegant prose that alcohol, like Dorian Gray (who appeared young and attractive until suddenly his true character is revealed as pernicious and destructive), is as dangerous as it always was.

(II:1) 98

Rubin, E., and C. Lieber. 1971. Alcoholism, alcohol and drugs. Science 172:1097-1102.

Data is presented supporting the general hypothesis that alcohol interferes with the metabolism and physiological disposal of other drugs, particularly barbiturates. Thus, in addition to its direct effects on the central nervous system, ethanol plays a role in the heightened sensitivity of inebriated persons.

(II:1) 99

Russell, M. A. 1971. Cigarette dependence: nature and classification. Brit. Med. J. 2:330-331.

A short article which summarizes current scientific evidence. Addiction to nicotine in cigarettes apparently follows the same physiological and psychological patterns as addiction to hard drugs.

(II:1) 100

Scott, J. M. 1964. The tea story.
    Funk and Wagnalls, New York.

    The cultural history of tea as
    a stimulant drug which is used
    as often as depressant alcoholic
    beverages within the same social
    context.

(II:1) 101

Tewari, S. 1971. Ethanol and brain protein
    synthesis. Brain Res. 26:469-474.

    Ethanol inhibits protein synthesis
    in the brain and therefore disrupts
    cognitive processes which are depen-
    dent upon unimpaired protein bio-
    synthetic cycles.

Section 2:   Stimulants

     a:   Amphetamines

(II:2) 102

Bradley, D. W., D. Joyce, E. H. Murphy,
    B. M. Nash, R. D. Porsoet, A. Sum-
    merfield, and W. A. Twyman. 1968.
    Amphetamine — barbiturate mixture:
    effects on the behavior of mice.
    Nature 220:187-188.

    The clinical impression that mixtures
    of amphetamines and barbiturates have
    psychoactive properties additional to
    those of the single constituents is
    supported by the results of experi-
    ments reported here.

(II:2) 103

Conwell, P. H. 1958. Amphetamine psychosis. Maudsley monog. No. 5 of the Institute of Psychiatry. Chapman and Hall, London.

A multidisciplinary survey of the subjective responses elicited by non-hallucinogenic amphetamine abuse. Detailed bibliographic material.

(II:2) 104

Galambos, E., A. L. Pfeifer, L. Gyorgy, and J. Molmar. 1967. Study on the excitation induced by amphetamine, codeine, and N-methyl-tryptamine. Psychopharmacologia 11:122-129.

The excitatory effects of a stimulant, a narcotic, and a hallucinogen are compared.

(II:2) 105

Hollister, L. E. 1969. An hallucinogenic amphetamine (DOM) in man. Psychopharmacologia 14:62-73.

An investigation of the physiological and psychological effects of one of the more potent hallucinogenic amphetamines. A DOM (STP) trip can last as long as three days, and evoke effects approximating those of LSD--depersonalization and synaesthesia (interchange of sensations: sight for sound, sound for touch, etc.). Note the discrepancy between Hollister's data on the duration of the drug's effect and figures reported by Snyder et al in 1967. A consensus seems to favor Hollister.

(II:2) 106

Leake, C. D. 1958. The amphetamines: their actions and uses. Charles C. Thomas, Springfield, Illinois.

A basic sourcebook on the physiology and biochemistry of amphetamine action. The hallucinogenic amphetamines are not discussed in detail.

(II:2) 107

Meyers, F. H., A. J. Rose, and D. E. Smith. 1968. Incidents involving the Haight-Ashbury population and some uncommonly used drugs. J. Psychedel. Drugs 1 (2): 136-146.

A study of the extent to which the hallucinogenic amphetamines (DOM, MDA, MMDA) and other "uncommon drugs" are used to imitate the sensations produced by the more widely-used psychotomimetics (drugs which mimic psychotic states).

(II:2) 108

Naranjo, D., A. T. Shulgin, and T. Sargent. 1967. Evaluation of 3, 4-methylenedioxy-amphetamine (MDA) as an adjunct to psychotherapy. Med. Parmacol. Exp. 17:359-364.

In a series of tests, doses of 150 mg. of MDA produced none of the perceptual alterations or depersonalization usually caused by related amphetamines and psychedelics. Instead, according to the authors, MDA elicited "heightened affect, emotional empathy, and access to feelings."

(II:2) 109

Russo, J. R. 1968. Amphetamine abuse.
Charles C. Thomas, Springfield,
Illinois.

This authoritative monograph deals with
the destructive effects of high doses
in amphetamine use. The author presents
detailed analyses of the personality
variable in the most serious of psychiatric consequences associated with
amphetamine abuse, such as auditory
and visual hallucinations with severe
paranoia.

(II:2) 110

Shulgin, A. T., S. Bunnell, and T. Sargent.
1961. The psychotomimetic properties of
3, 4, 5-trimethoxyamphetamine. Nature
189:1011-1012.

Although TMA was first synthesized in
1947, its effects remained largely un-
explored until this time. TMA is
twice as active as mescaline and elicits
similar auditory and tactile sensations
when administered at low doses. Higher
doses cause antisocial responses including anger, hostility, and megalo-
manic euphoria.

(II:2) 111

Shulgin, A. T. 1964. 3-Methoxy-4, 5-methylene-
dioxyamphetamine, a new psychotomimetic
agent. Nature 201:1120-1121.

MMDA (as it is commonly known) is three
times more potent than mescaline in
human subjects. The effects of MMDA,
like those of TMA, are hallucinogenic
and allow complete recall. Shulgin
synthesized this amphetamine from my-
risticin, another essential oil found
in nutmeg.

(II:2) 112

Shulgin, A. T., T. Sargent, and C. Naranjo. 1969. Structure-activity relationships of one-ring psychotomimetics. Nature 221:537-541.

A report on the biological testing of over 40 psychotomimetic amphetamines on human subjects, including details on the chemical syntheses, physiological doses, and psychological effects of the compounds tested compared to those of a known hallucinogen, mescaline. Shulgin is a leading experimenter in this field, and most of the literature on the subject has been produced from his laboratory.

(II:2) 113

Smith, D. E., ed. 1969. Speed kills: a review of amphetamine drug abuse. J. Psychedel. Drugs 2(2). A symposium volume.

A series of papers by psychiatrists and physicians, practicing mostly in California, presenting especially interesting information on the hallucinogenic amphetamines. Detailed bibliographies on each topic are included.

(II:2) 114

Snyder, S. H., L. Faillace, and L. Hollister. 1967. 2, 5-dimethoxy-4-methyl-amphetamine (STP); a new hallucinogenic drug. Science 158:669-670.

The effects of this widely used amphetamine are assessed in normal control volunteers. In low doses--below 3 milligrams per individual--STP produced mild euphoria. In higher doses, STP "may cause pronounced hallucinogenic effects lasting 8 hours and similar to those produced by LSD, mescaline, and psilocybin."

(II:2) 115

Van Rossum, J. M. 1970. Mode of action of psychomotor stimulant drugs. Int. Rev. Neurobiol. 12:307-383.

A critical review of the research and clinical literature on the pharmacodynamic and toxicological effects of amphetamines and related compounds.

(II:2) 116

Weiss, B., and V. G. Laties. 1962. Enhancement of human performance by caffeine and the amphetamines. Pharmacol. Rev. 14:1-36.

Notes 118 references about these stimulants, including methedrine, benzedrine, and dexedrine.

b: Cocaine

(II:2) 117

Adriani, J. 1960. The clinical pharmacology of local anesthetics. Clin. Pharmacol. Therap. 1:645-673.

Cocaine is widely used as a local anesthetic and thus acute poisoning from cocaine is not rare. The symptoms are 1) enhanced reflexes, 2) anxiety, 3) restlessness, and in terminal cases, 4) delirium and death. This review article also discusses the clinical application of several cocaine analogues.

(II:2) 118

Bejerot, N. 1970. A comparison of the effects of cocaine and synthetic central stimulants. Brit. J. Addic. 65:35-37.

From a survey of the literature the author concludes that the effects of synthetic stimulants (amphetamines and related compounds) "in all essentials resemble cocainism," a state characterized by euphoria, psychic dependence, restlessness, talkativeness, pleasurable physical exhilaration and raised blood pressure.

(II:2) 119

Blyer-Prieto, H. 1965. Coca leaf and cocaine addiction: some historical notes. Canad. Med. Ass. J. 93:700-704.

    Sociological and historical information on the uses of coca leaves as a stimulant and of cocaine as a local anesthetic.

(II:2) 120

Gramer-Doyeux, M. 1962. Some sociological aspects of the problem of cocaism. Bull. Narcotics 14(4):1-16.

    The author asserts that cocaism--the habit of chewing coca leaves--is the result of a series of unfavorable social, economic, cultural, and hygienic factors in South America. A lengthy bibliography.

(II:2) 121

Hanna, J. M. 1970. The effects of coca chewing on exercise in the Quechua of Peru. Human Biol. 42(1):1-11.

    The supposition that cocaine-containing leaves increase working capacity and endurance of hunger in users is supported by physiological data.

(II:2) 122

Kalyanpur, S. G., and B. E. Ryman. 1966. Some effects of local anesthetics on cell metabolism. Biochem. Pharmacol. 15:691-701.

    Contains a discussion of cocaine's biochemical action; the most important local action being its ability to block nerve conduction.

## Section 3: Tranquilizers

(II:3) 123

Adams, E. 1958. Barbiturates. Sci. Am. 190(1):60-64.

Short, readable, and practically still up-to-date. Treats the physiological and clinical aspects of barbiturate use.

(II:3) 124

Beecher, H. K. 1957. The measurement of pain. Pharmacol. Rev. 9:59-297.

An exhaustive review of pain-killers and tranquilizers. Principal laboratory and clinical studies are described with reference to 687 publications. Information offered here is also reviewed by the same author in entries 44, 45, and 46 of Chapter I.

(II:3) 125

Bradley, P. B. 1963. Phenothiazine derivatives. Pages 417-77 in Root, W. S. and F. G. Hoffman, eds. Physiological pharmacology. Academic Press, New York.

A sixty-page review on the mode of action, clinical application and biological effects of these widely-used major tranquilizers. A definitive bibliography.

(II:3) 126

Chambers, C. D. 1969. Barbiturate-sedative abuse: a study of prevalence among narcotic abusers. Int. J. Addict. 4: 45-57.

Heroin addicts are known in many instances to be partial towards barbiturates as a second drug. The author traces the parallel between the psychic states produced by these two kinds of drugs and concludes they are more closely related than would be the corresponding psychic states produced by stimulants or psychedelics.

(II:3) 127

Conney, A. H. 1971. Pharmacological implications of microsomal enzyme induction. Pharmacol. Rev. 19:317.

This article provides an exhaustive review of the effects of drugs, particularly the tranquilizers, on the enzyme systems which all higher organisms use to dispose of noxious chemicals. Here is a classic example of how drugs that "affect" the "mind" can also affect the "body" by a completely unrelated biochemical mechanism.

(II:3) 128

Devenyi, P. 1971. Barbiturate abuse and addiction and their relationship to alcohol and alcoholism. Can. Med. Ass. J. 104:215-218.

The article documents the use of depressants by alcoholics. Forty-three references to the current literature are included.

(II:3) 129

Dixon, A. St. J., B. K. Martin, M. J. H. Smith, and P. H. N. Wood, eds. 1963. Salicylates: an international symposium. J & A Churchill, Ltd., London.

A comprehensive, multidisciplinary review, considered still current.

(II:3) 130

Domino, E. F. 1962. Human pharmacology of tranquilizing drugs. Clin. Pharmacol. Therap. 3:599-664.

A general review covering studies on barbiturates and non-barbiturate sedatives, and hypnotics.

(II:3) 131

Doty, B. A., and L. A. Doty. 1964. Effect of age and chlorpromazine on memory consolidation. J. Comp. Physiol. Psychiat. 57:331-334.

The effects of a tranquilizer upon learning and memory in rats. Chlorpromazine (thorazine) seems to inhibit the memory processes.

(II:3) 132

Essig, C. F. 1964. Addiction to non-barbiturate sedatives and tranquilizing drugs. Clin. Pharmacol. Therap. 5:334-343.

Discusses addiction to such drugs as Nodular, Doriden, Meisedin and others.

(II:3) 133

Gates, M. 1966. Analgesic drugs. Sci. Am. 215(5):131-136.

The chemistry of pain-killers modelled after morphine, but without addictive side-effects. Structure-activity relationships are explained intelligibly.

(II:3) 134

Goldberg, L. 1961. Alcohol, tranquilizers, and hangover. Quart. J. Stud. Alc. Suppl. 1:37-56.

A detailed analysis of the use of tranquilizers in treatment of the symptoms of alcoholism.

(II:3) 135

Goldberg, M. E., A. A. Manian, and D. H. Fron. 1967. A comparative study of certain pharmacologic responses following acute and chronic administrations of chlordiazepoxide. Life Sci. 6:481-491.

The physiological and behavioral consequences of repeated overuse of Librium.

(II:3) 136

Grisolia, S., I. Santos, and J. Mendelson. 1968. Inactivating enzymes by aspirin and salicylate. Nature 219:1252.

Although aspirin (acetylsalicylic acid) and related compounds are generally considered to be "harmless drugs," the researchers note that these compounds have a profound effect on nitrogen metabolism. The experimental evidence indicates that the drugs enhance protein breakdown and therefore cause significant increases in the concentration of non-protein nitrogen compounds in living systems.

(II:3) 137

Gorss, M., and L. A. Greenberg. 1948. The salicylates: a critical bibliographic review. Hillhouse Press, New Haven.

A survey of the older literature (4093 references).

(II:3) 138

Hoffeld, D. R., R. L. Webster, and J. McNew. 1967. Adverse effects on offspring of tranquilizing drugs during pregnancy. Nature 215:182-183.

The general conclusion from the result of this study is that the administration of tranquilizing drugs to gravid rats produces adverse health and learning effects in the offspring. Meprobamate (Equanil, Miltown), chlorpromazine (thorazine), and reserpine (Serpasil), and other drugs used had varying adverse effects, depending on the period of administration, and none was uniformly deleterious.

(II:3) 139

Isbell, H., and H. F. Fraser. 1950. Addiction to analgesics and barbiturates. Pharmacol. Rev. 2:355-397.

General information covering almost five decades of literature.

(II:3) 140

Kalant, H., A. E. LeBlanc, R. J. Gibbins. 1971. Tolerance to, and dependence on, some non-opiate psychotropic drugs. Pharmacol. Rev. 23:135-191.

This review covers information taken from 402 research publications on the subject of addiction to barbiturates, phenothiazines, sedative hypnotics, stimulants, and hallucinogens. Information on the metabolism and mode of action of these drugs is also included along with extensive definitions of terminology used to describe the addiction process.

(II:3) 141

Kehoe, M. J. 1971. Major tranquilizers. South. Med. J. 64:403-410.

A medical review with 20 references to the current literature on reserpine, phenothiazine, phenothiazine-like drugs, and lithium carbonate.

(II:3) 142

Kyogoku, Y., R. C. Lord, and H. Rich. 1968. Specific hydrogen bonding of barbiturates to adenine derivatives. Nature 218:69-72.

Selective hydrogen bonding is one of the most important forces in the process of biological organization at the molecular level. It is by this process, for example, that the double helix of DNA is held together. Barbiturates (phenobarbital, secobarbital, thiopental and others) have been shown to attach themselves to adenine, a component of DNA, and therefore may play some role in altering the shape of DNA molecules and the function of genes. To date, these results have not been verified in living organisms.

(II:3) 143

Lasagna, L. 1954. A comparison of hypnotic agents. J. Pharmacol. Expt. Ther. 111: 9-20.

A general review of mostly clinical information about such drugs as Equanil, Librium, and Valium.

(II:3) 144

Mendelson, J., D. Wexler, P. H. Leiderman, and P. Solomon. 1957. A study of addiction to nonethyl alcohols and other poisonous compounds. Quart. J. Stud. Alcohol. 18:561-580.

Includes discussions of the effects of Dormison (methylpentynol) and Placidyl (ethchlorvinol) and other sedatives and hypnotics.

(II:3) 145

Norton, P. R. E. 1971. Some endocrinological aspects of barbiturate dependence. Brit. J. Pharmacol. 41: 317-330.

Like many other drugs, barbiturates affect a variety of tissues and organs other than those in the nervous system. The author discusses a case in point: his experiments indicate that rats dependent on barbiturates have larger thyroid and adrenal glands, a larger liver, smaller gonads and larger secondary sex organs than untreated animals.

(II:3) 146

Onishi, S. I., and H. M. McConnell. 1965.
Interaction of the radical ion of
chlorpromazine with deoxyribonucleic
acid. J. Amer. Chem. Soc. 87:2293.

An *in vitro* study of the chemical
reactivity of chlorpromazine. The drug
forms complexes with DNA, the heredity-
governing molecule, and may thus cause
genetic damage in living organisms; but
this possibility has not yet been demonstrated *in vivo*.

(II:3) 147

Palfai, T., and J. M. Cornell. 1968.
Effect of drugs on the consolidation
of classically conditioned fear.
J. Comp. Physiol. Psychiat. 66:584-
589.

According to current hypotheses,
consolidation or permanent storage
of an experience in memory requires
some period of neural activity ini-
tiated by the experience to be remembered. Because the tranquilizer Metra-
zol depresses neural activity, it was
found to produce amnesia when administered to rats, shortly after they had
been trained to perform a specific task.

(II:3) 148

Sternbach, L. H. 1971. 1, 4-benzodiazepines.
Chemistry and some aspects of the
structure activity relationship.
Angew. Chem. Int. Ed. Eng. 10:30-43.

A critical appraisal of the biochemical
mechanisms by which drugs like Librium
and Valium exert their specific tranquilizing or antipsychotic effect.
Emphasis is placed on the relationships
between the chemical structure and
biological activity of this class of
drugs.

## Section 4: Narcotics

(II:4) 149

Adriani, J., ed. 1964. Narcotics and narcotic antagonists. Charles C. Thomas, Springfield, Illinois.

A survey in anthology form of the chemistry, pharmacology, and applications of certain narcotic painkillers in anesthesiology and obstetrics. Several essays in this volume address themselves to the procedural difficulties encountered by clinicians, particularly when confronted with the task of counteracting the effects of routinely used narcotics.

(II:4) 150

Austin, B. L. 1970. Sad nun at Synanon. Holt, Rinehart and Winston, New York.

Another account of the rehabilitation process for heroin addicts at the Synanon Foundation. A woman's treatment of the subject of identity crises among addicts, and their progressive resolution. (Compare with Yablonsky, Ref. #178).

(II:4) 151

Boyd, P. 1970. Heroin addiction in adolescents. J. Psychosom. Res. 14:295-301.

A statistical survey along with speculations as to the causes of narcotic addiction in youths under 18.

(II:4) 152

Denton, J. E., and H. K. Beecher. 1949.
New analgesics II. A clinical appraisal of the narcotic power of methadone and its isomers. III. A comparison of the side effects of morphine, methadone, and methadone's powers in man. J. Amer. Med. Assoc. 141:1146-1153.

Two papers describing the first thorough studies on methadone more than a decade before it began to receive attention as an agent for the rehabilitation of heroin addicts.

(II:4) 153

Dole, V. P., and M. Nyswander. 1965.
A medical treatment for diacetylmorphine. Heroin addiction--a clinical test with methadone hydrochloride. J. Amer. Med. Assoc. 198:646-650.

Dr. Nyswander has been influential in gaining professional acceptance of methadone as a viable form of replacement therapy in heroin addiction. The article reports the results of a typical clinical trial.

(II:4) 154

Encyclopedia Britannica. 1911. 11th ed.
Opium. Vol. XX:130-137.

One of the best historical reviews for information on the botanical origins and primitive uses of the drug, also reflecting Victorian and Edwardian attitudes.

(II:4) 155

Fraser, H. F., G. D. Van Horn, W. R. Martin, A. B. Wolbach, and H. Isbell. 1961. Methods for evaluating addiction liability. (a) 'attitude' of opiate addicts toward opiate-like drugs. (b) a short-term 'direct' addiction test. J. Pharmacol. Exp. Therap. 133:371-387.

An important contribution to the methodology of the study of drug addiction. The authors define the necessary subjective parameters that must be considered in investigations of the subject.

(II:4) 156

Goldstein, A. 1972. Heroin addiction and the role of methadone and its treatment. Arch. Gen. Psychiat. 26:291-298.

Dr. Goldstein, who is on the staff of the Addiction Research Laboratory at Stanford, has put together one of the few existing short and useful clinical reviews of the vast literature on heroin addiction. He discusses the physiologically pleasurable effects of heroin and the nature of tolerance and physical dependence, and then explains how methadone works to "stabilize" heroin dependence by suppressing withdrawal symptoms. The essay includes 35 citations to literature from 1967-1971.

(II:4) 157

Hesse, E. 1946. Narcotics and drug addiction. Philosophical Library, New York.

Although as a general exposition on the subject of opiates, it is quite out of date, the book is cited for its colorful historical references to opiates, cocaine and marihuana and other psychoactive drugs such as aphrodisiacs. Lengthy personal accounts compiled by the author are included.

(II:4) 158

Kolb, L. 1925. Pleasure and deterioration from narcotic addiction. Ment. Hyg. 9:699-724.

Kolb takes issue with the myth perhaps most widely propagated by de Quincey's *Confessions of an English Opium Eater*, that opiates produce euphoria. He states categorically as a result of his own researches that "only in rare instances, if at all, does anyone except the emtoionally unstable, the psychopath, or the neurotic experience pleasure from morphine."

(II:4) 159

Kritikos, P. G., and S. P. Papdaki. 1967. The history of the poppy and of opium and their expansion in antiquity in the eastern Mediterranean area. Pts. I, I:. Bull. Narcotics 19(3):17-88; 19(4):5-10.

Classical sources, archaeological discoveries in Greece, numismatic and etymological evidence attest to the widespread use of opiates in classical antiquity.

(II:4) 160

Larner, J., and R. Tefferteller. 1964. The addict in the street. Grove Press, New York.

The phenomenon of addiction can be studied on two planes, from the cerebral point of view of the research psychiatrist or from the visceral point of view of the man on the street. The latter sets the tone and the pace for this anthology of transcribed interviews with 13 addicts. The book is designed to sensitize the reader to the human needs of the chronic drug user.

(II:4) 161

Lasagna, L. 1964. Chemical evaluation of morphine and its substitutes as analgesics. Pharmacol. Rev. 16:47-83.

A review of the quantitative data available on the clinical efficacy and safety of narcotic pain-killers. 160 references.

(II:4) 162

Lasagna, L., J. M. von Felsinger, and H. K. Beecher. 1955. Drug induced mood changes in man. I. Observations on healthy subjects, chronically ill patients, and "past addicts". J. Amer. Med. Assoc. 157:1006-1020.

A study confirming many of Kolb's earlier observations. The majority of subjects treated found first exposures to morphine and heroin unpleasant, and such data implies according to the authors that an abnormal psychological state or physiological condition must preexist in order for the drugs to function as euphoriants.

(II:4) 163

Moscow, A. 1968. Merchants of heroin. Dial Press, New York.

When, where, and how: a searching presentation of business in the underworld.

(II:4) 164

National Research Council. 1941. Report of the committee on drug addiction, 1921-1941. National Research Council, Washington, D.C.

Collected reprints of chemical, pharmacological and clinical research papers on opiates and opiate derivatives. More than 1500 pages of data.

(II:4) 165

Neuberg, R. 1970. Drug dependence and pregnancy: a review of the problems and their management. J. Obstet. Gynaecol. Brit. Common. 77:1117-1122.

A review of the potential dangers to both the mother and the fetus presented by addiction to heroin or to other drugs.

(II:4) 166

Nichols, J. R. 1965. How opiates change behavior. Sci. Am. 212(2):80-90.

A model experiment. Nichols has noted that rats trained to administer morphine to themselves become addicted, whereas those that receive the drug passively do not. Presumably, addiction is a function of the frequency of opiate intake.

(II:4) 167

Pharmacology Society Symposium. 1970. New concepts and approaches to the study of drug dependence and addiction. Fed. Proc. 29:2-32.

The symposium presents five up-to-date review papers on the following topics pertaining to opiate addiction: 1) Psychological approaches to opiate dependence and self-administration by laboratory animals. 2) Stimulant self-administration by animals: some comparisons with opiate self-administration. 3) Pharmacological redundancy as an adaptive mechanism in the development of tolerance. 4) Central neurohumoral systems involved with narcotic agonists and antagonists.

(II:4) 168

Ramirez, E. 1968. The existential approach to the management of character disorders with special reference to narcotic drug addiction. Rev. Exist. Psychol. Psychiat. 8:43-53.

Guidelines for the rehabilitation of addicts. The author emphasizes the notion that the setting in which the rehabilitation process is to take place must be carefully constructed and controlled. The concept of a therapeutic community is also proposed.

(II:4) 169

Reynolds, A. K., and L. O. Randall. 1957. Morphine and allied drugs. University of Toronto Press, Toronto.

A definitive sourcebook describing the research and findings reported in more than 1600 publications on opiates.

(II:4) 170

Steinberg, H., ed. 1969. Scientific basis of drug dependence: a symposium. Churchill, London.

Papers mostly about opiates, presenting a comprehensive view of the subject as it is currently understood, from a symposium held in April, 1968 under the sponsorship of the British Pharmacological Society. The writing is generally quite academic.

(II:4) 171

Vaillant, G. E. 1966. A 12-year follow-up of New York narcotic addicts: some social and psychiatric characteristics. Arch. Gen. Psychiat. 15:599-609.

Sociological correlations, behavioral patterns, and types of subjective response are discussed.

(II:4) 172

Vaillant, G. E. 1966. Twelve-year follow-up of New York narcotic addicts, II: the natural history of chronic disease. New. Eng. J. Med. 275:1282-1288.

The second part of one of the few available long-range studies, presenting data from carefully followed case histories. Discusses general trends.

(II:4) 173

Vaillant, G. E. 1970. The natural history of
   drug addiction. Sem. Psychiat. 2:486-498.

   Dr. Vaillant reviews the predisposing
   factors of addiction. "Perhaps no mental
   illness," he argues, "is more a product of
   its social setting than addiction to narcotics. Drugs depend both for their desirabil-
   ity and for their effect on the milieu in
   which they are taken. Both the ritualisation
   and the modes of drug taking depend upon and
   usually create a sub-culture. Thus, in part,
   the natural history of drug addiction is
   like that of society; it must be rewritten
   every few years." The information in this
   remarkable essay updates previous publication by the author. 27 references accompany
   the text.

(II:4) 174

Von Felsinger, J. M., L. Lasagna, and H. K.
   Beecher. 1955. Drug induced mood changes
   in man: II. Personality and reaction to
   drugs. J. Amer. Med. Assoc. 157:1113-1119.

   A description and analysis of the subjective responses reported in Part I of
   this article. (Ref. 126)

(II:4) 175

Walsh, J. 1970. Methadone and heroin addiction:
   rehabilitation without a "cure." Science
   168:684-686.

   "Faced with the literally hopeless situation of so many heroin addicts," writes
   the author, "some partisans of methadone
   treatment endow methadone with almost
   magical properties, and journalists have
   tended to follow their lead." Walsh con-
   tinues with a discussion of the pros and
   cons of methadone in the detoxification or
   "withdrawal" of heroin addicts. Current
   FDA attitudes toward the drug are also
   described.

(II:4) 176

Weeks, J. R. 1964. Experimental narcotic addiction. Sci. Am. 210(3):46-52.

By allowing addicted monkeys and rats to give themselves intravenous injections at will, the authors have studied some of the motivational factors affecting the voluntary intake of opiates (morphine, codeine, and heroin).

(II:4) 177

Weppuer, R. S., and M. A. Agar. 1971. Immediate precursors to heroin addiction. J. Health Soc. Behav. 12:10-18.

The authors examine the "stepping stone" hypothesis so often invoked as an explanation for heroin addiction. They conclude from a statistical study that there is no single immediate precursor to heroin addiction (such as marihuana, amphetamine or barbiturate abuse), but that the precursor drugs differ when different social groupings are considered.

(II:4) 178

Yablonsky, L. 1965. The tunnel back: Synanon. MacMillan, New York.

A description of the rehabilitation of heroin addicts at the Synanon Foundation. A point of view on the restoration of addicts' sense of self-identity both as individuals and as members of a community.

Section 5: Psychedelics

a: LSD and related drugs

(II:5) 179

Aaronson, B. S. 1967. LSD: experimental findings. Int. J. Parapsychol. 9: 86-90.

    The author traces the relationship between hypnotic states and drug induced psychedelic states.

(II:5) 180

Aaronson, B., and H. Osmond, eds. 1970. Psychedelics. Anchor-Doubleday, Garden City, New York.

    The most recent study of the uses and consequences of psychedelics, a book whose bulk is bracketed by powerful introductory and concluding chapters. In between, distinguished essayists and authorities discuss the following topics: the nature of the psychedelic experience; the effects of psychedelics on religious experience, psychedelic effects on mental function, non-drug analogues to the psychedelic state, and sociology of psychedelics in the current scene. An extensive bibliography serves particularly well as a guide to information on the role of the psychedelic state in the arts and philosophy.

(II:5) 181

Alpert, R., and S. Cohen. 1966. LSD. The New American Library, New York.

    A question-and-answer discussion between Richard Alpert (Baba Ram Dass) and Sidney Cohen, emphasizing the nature of the LSD experience and the potential influence of the drug on society.

(II:5) 182

Amarel, M., and F. E. Cheek. 1965. Some
 effects of LSD-25 on verbal communication.
 J. Abnor. Psychol. 70:453-456.

 Evidence is presented specifically
 concerning the effect of LSD and related psychedelics on the user's ability
 to express himself coherently and effectively.

(II:5) 183

Bakker, C. B., and F. Amini. 1961. Observations
 on the psychotomimetic effect of sernyl.
 Comp. Psychiat. 2:269-280.

 Sernyl (phencyclidine) has been used widely
 as a main ingredient in "street" preparations
 passed off most often as mescaline, MDA, and
 sometimes even as LSD. The drug was developed
 originally as an anesthetic. It causes
 muscular incoordination, double vision,
 dizziness, and near maniac states of excitation. In this research study, Bakker
 and Amini further point out that the drug serves
 to worsen whatever psychotic symptoms its users
 may have.

(II:5) 184

Blacker, K. H., R. T. Jones, G. C. Stone,
 and D. Pfefferbaum. 1968. Chronic users
 of LSD: the "acidheads." Amer. J.
 Psychiat. 125:341-351.

 Studies based on a wide sampling of
 "acidheads" in San Francisco, documenting
 their borderline reality contact, vague-
 ness, lethargy and incipient schizophrenia.

(II:5) 185

Blewett, D. B. 1963. Psychedelic drugs in
 parapsychological research. Int. J.
 Parapsychol. 5.

 An essay on the uses of LSD in extrasensory perception research. This review
 article is recommended for the citations
 which amply cover the existing literature.

(II:5) 186

Blum, R., et al. Utopiates: the use and
users of LSD-25. Atherton, New York.

An anthology of writings on various
aspects of LSD use--history, pharmacology,
social implications, religion, legal controls,
etc. Of particular interest are the articles
on the short-lived International Federation
of Internal Freedom (IFIF) psychedelic
training center set up by Timothy Leary
in Zihuatanejo, Mexico. Recommended by
many reviewers, including the editors of
Psychedelic Review.

(II:5) 187

Caldwell, W. V. 1968. LSD Psychotherapy.
Grove Press, New York.

A treatment of the history and practice
of psychedelic psychotherapy, but not as
detailed as other review volumes. A notable contribution for the description and
classification of basic universal fantasies
manifested in persons under the influence
of hallucinogens.

(II:5) 188

Campaigne, E., and D. R. Knapp. 1971.
Structural analogs of lysergic acid.
J. Pharmaceut. Sci. 60:809-813.

A literature survey with 57 citations.
The authors describe syntheses of over
fifty structural analogues of LSD and
compare their biological activity to that
of the parent molecule. In several cases
they find that the derivatives proved to
be more potent effectors of neural processes than the parent compound.

(II:5) 189

Cavanna, R., and E. Servadis. 1964. ESP experiments with LSD-25 and psilocybin: a methodological approach. Parapsychology Foundation, New York.

A meticulous analysis of why these experiments failed, offering guidelines for the design of future tests. An interesting book, if only for its methodological acrobatics.

(II:5) 190

Debold, R. C., and R. C. Leaf. 1967. LSD, man and society. Wesleyan University Press, Middletown, Conn.

An anthology covering a variety of topics, including "Motivational Patterns in LSD Usage", "Social and Legal Aspects of LSD Usage", and "The Pharmacology of LSD". More generally scholarly in tone than Solomon's. (Ref. 203)

(II:5) 191

Eells, K. 1968. LSD. Institute of Technology Press, Pasadena.

A multiphasic text, presenting balanced opinions and serving as a general reference for scientific and sociological information.

(II:5) 192

Fadiman, J., W. W. Harman, R. H. McKim, R. E. Mogar, and M. J. Stolaroff. 1965. Psychedelic agents in creative problem solving. Institute for Psychedelic Research of San Francisco State College, San Francisco.

The performance of volunteers under the influence of LSD and other psychedelics compared with that of control individuals in a number of experiments suggests that psychedelic drugs may, in many cases, elicit novel approaches to problem solving.

(II:5) 193

Fogel, S., and A. Hoffer. 1962. The use of hypnosis to interrupt and to reproduce an LSD-25 experience. J. Clin. Exp. Psych. 23:11-16.

The authors underscore the intimate relationship between psychedelic states and parallel, non-drug psychic conditions.

(II:5) 194

Hoffer, A. and H. Osmond. 1968. The hallucinogens. Academic Press, New York.

Osmond and his co-writers almost invariably produce work of high quality. This definitive study offers scientific facts as well as historical description. An essential bibliographical sourcebook, but difficult to obtain except in libraries.

(II:5) 195

Klee, G. 1963. Lysergic acid diethylamide (LSD-25) and ego functions. Arch. Gen. Psychiat. 8:461-474.

About LSD and its effect on the user's conception of himself. Under the influence of psychedelics the ego is said to both shrink and expand to varying degrees. Dr. Klee's article is one frequently cited as an authoritative study of the subject.

(II:5) 196

Kobler, J. 1963. The dangerous magic of LSD. Saturday Evening Post, 2 Nov:30-40.

Represenative of the sense of awe with which journalists regarded LSD in the early sixties.

(II:5) 197

Lennard, H., M. E. Jarvik, and H. A. Abramson. 1956. Lysergic acid diethylamide (LSD-25): XII. A preliminary statement of its effects upon interpersonal communication. J. Psychol. 41:185-198.

Results of the experiments reported have led to the conclusion that in general LSD impedes verbal communication more often than not, although it enhances the effectiveness of the non-verbal component in interpersonal relationships established during use of the psychedelic.

(II:5) 198

Lindgren, J. E., G. G. Hammer, R. Hessling, and B. Holmstedt. 1969. The chemical identity of "hog"--a new hallucinogen. Amer. J. Pharmacol. 141:86-90.

The widespread use of Sernyl (phencyclidine) as a substitute for popular hallucinogens is described in this scientific expose of one of the more dangerous deceptions on the illicit drug market.

(II:5) 199

Meyer, R. E. 1969. Adverse reactions to hallucinogenic drugs. Public Health Serv. Pub. No. 180. Dep. of Health, Education and Welfare, U.S. Government Printing Office, Washington, D.C.

A transcript of a 1967 conference, a bibliography of 70 references to articles on possible genetic after-effects of hallucinogenic and other drugs, and reprints of several papers in this area.

(II:5) 200

National Library of Medicine Literature
    Searches. 1968. Adverse effects of
    LSD. Dep. of Health, Education and
    Welfare, U.S. Government Printing
    Office, Washington, D.C.

A bibliography (L.S. No. 24-68) citing
112 references from January 1964 to
August 1968.

(II:5) 201

National Library of Medicine Literature
    Searches. 1968. Effect of hallucinogens
    on man. Dep. of Health, Education and
    Welfare, U.S. Government Printing Office,
    Washington, D.C.

A bibliography (L.S. No. 30-68) citing
303 references from January 1966 to
August 1968.

(II:5) 202

Pollard, J. C., L. Uhr, and E. Stern. 1965.
    Drugs and phantasy. The effects of
    LSD, psilocybin and sernyl on college
    students. Little, Brown and Company,
    Boston.

Actual transcribed data from controlled
experiments with two psychedelics and
one anesthetic (sernyl) are presented as
part of lengthy firsthand accounts.
The studies were conducted at the University of Michigan Health Research
Institute. Perhaps the most important
findings presented in this report relate
to the effects of supportive environments on the magnitude of a psychedelic

experience. Subjects who were isolated
from auditory, visual and tactile stimuli
failed to register the usual responses
under the influence of psychedelics.

(II:5) 203

Solomon, D. 1964. LSD: the consciousness-expanding drug. G. P. Putnam's Sons, New York.

Articles on a variety of topics related to LSD by contributors such as Leary, Huxley, Osmond, Watts and Burroughs. Heavily biased in favor of psychedelics. Recommended highly by the editors of Psychedelic Review for its philosophical and scientific viewpoints.

(II:5) 204

U. S. Public Health Service. Bibliography on psychotomimetics, 1943-66. Dep. of Health, Education and Welfare, U.S. Government Printing Office, Washington, D.C.

Most of the references in this annotated bibliography concern LSD, but information on mescaline and psilocybin is also included. Annotations are generally very detailed, and are, in some cases, several paragraphs long.

b: Mescaline, mushrooms and molds

(II:5) 205

Aberle, D. F. 1966. The peyote religion among the Navaho. Aldine Publishing Co., Chicago.

A sociological and historical survey devoted especially to Navaho culture.

(II:5) 206

Bergman, R. L. 1971. Navajo peyote use: its
   apparent safety. Amer. J. Psychiat. 128:
   695-699.

   Although the Navajo Indians consume
   significant quantities of peyote, they
   suffer few emotional disturbances caused
   by similar drugs, because the feelings
   evoked by the drug experience are chan-
   neled by church belief and practice into
   ego-strengthening directions.

(II:5) 207

Farnsworth, N. R. 1968. Hallucinogenic plants.
   Science. 162:1086-1092.

   A straightforward pharmacological survey with structural formulae and dosage
   data for the major hallucinogens.

(II:5) 208

Kapadia, G. J., and M. B. E. Fayez. 1970.
   Peyote constituents: chemistry, bio-
   genesis, and biological effects. J.
   Pharmaceut. Sci. 59:1699-1727.

   A key reference on the subject of peyote.
   In this review article are discussed the
   historical backgrounds of peyote use, the
   chemistry of over fifty constituents of
   the peyote button (along with a survey of
   synthetic schemes), their biosynthesis,
   and their biological effects. 435 references
   are cited.

(II:5) 209

Keeler, M. H. 1965. The effects of psilocybin
   on a test of afterimage perception.
   Psychopharmacologia 8:131-139.

   A study on the effect of the psychedelic
   as a mediator in the formation of visual
   color patterns.

(II:5) 210

Kluver, H. 1966. Mescal and mechanisms of hallucination. University of Chicago Press, Chicago.

An excellent short book on the psychological as well as psychic workings of mescaline, lucidly covering scientific aspects of the subject, with occasional quotations from Baudelaire. A good bibliography and index.

(II:5) 211

La Barre, W. 1960. Twenty years of peyote studies. Curr. Anthropol. 1:45-60.

Useful as a bibliographic guide.

(II:5) 212

La Barre, W. 1964. The peyote cult. The Shoestring Press, Hamden, Conn.

A thorough history of peyote use among the American Indians, including an extensive bibliography.

(II:5) 213

Leary, T. R., G. H. Litwin, and R. Metzner. 1963. Reactions to psilocybin administered in a supportive environment. J. Nerv. Ment. Dis. 137:561-573.

Psilocybin's effects compare to those of LSD, especially when it is taken in a setting that re-enforces that notion. In non-supportive environments the psychic response to psilocybin appears to be attenuated.

(II:5) 214

McGlothlin, W. H. 1965. Hallucinogen drugs: a perspective with special reference to peyote and cannabis. Psychedel. Rev. 6: 16-57.

A review article on the historical uses of the two drugs. McGlothlin faithfully reports both favorable and unfavorable information, citing 122 references.

(II:5) 215

Metzner, R., G. Litwin, and G. M. Weil. 1965. The relations of expectation and mood to psilocybin reactions: a questionnaire study. Psychedel. Rev. 5:3-39.

Among 82 subjects tested, subjective experiences were found to vary according to pre-trial expectations. The elaborate questionnaire is reproduced.

(II:5) 216

Pennington, W. 1963. The Tarahumar of Mexico-- their environment and material culture. University of Utah Press, Salt Lake City.

A multiphasic study of the peyote worshippers of northern Mexico. According to the author, the Tarahumar Indians have fashioned their rituals, customs and folklore upon the premise that when Father Sun left earth to dwell in the heavens, he left the mescal button on earth to mollify man's pain and woe.

(II:5) 217

Puharich, A. 1959. The sacred mushroom.
    Doubleday, Garden City.

Amanita muscaria (fly agaric, soma) is central to ancient Egyptian culture and religion, according to Puharich's interpretation of certain hieroglyphs. Presented as an account, in the first person, of how the author came upon the "key to the door of eternity."

(II:5) 218

Schultes, R. E. 1969, 1970. The plant kingdom and hallucinogens. Bull Narcotics (Pt. I) 21(3):3-16; (Pt. II) 21(4):15-27; (Pt. III) 22(1):25-53.

This series is highly recommended. It covers the history of ethnopharmacology with particular regard to the botanical origins and uses of all known hallucinogens.

(II:5) 219

Schultes, R. E. 1969. Hallucinogens of plant origin. Science 163:245-254.

The same subject as Farnsworth's (Ref. #207), but with more emphasis on cultural aspects than on chemistry.

(II:5) 220

Schultes, R. E., and A. Hofmann. 1972. The botany and chemistry of hallucinogens. Charles C. Thomas, Springfield, Illinois.

An extensive and comprehensive scholarly survey, entirely up-to-date, particularly on the cultural and historical dimensions of hallucinogen "chemistry." This book serves well as an encyclopedia in the subject.

(II:5) 221

Slotkin, J. 1956. The peyote religion.
    Free Press, Glencoe, Illinois.

   An anthropological study of the
   Native American Church, a religion
   centered around the use of the mescal
   button.

(II:5) 222

Unger, S. M. 1963. Mescaline, LSD, psilocybin,
    and personality change. Psychiatry 26:111-125.

   The subjective effects of the three psychedelics are compared in terms of what they
   do to the user's character and vision of
   himself. The author also presents a
   critical evaluation of similar studies
   on this matter.

(II:5) 223

Wasson, R. G. 1963. The hallucinogenic fungi
    of Mexico. Psychedel. Rev. 1:27-42.

   An inquiry into the origins of the
   religious idea among primitive people.
   Wasson deals mostly with Mexican civili-
   zations, but also discusses, for comparative purooses, the Eleusinian Mysteries
   of ancient Greece.

(II:5) 224

Wasson, R. G. 1969. Soma: Divine mushroom of
    immortality. Harcourt, Brace & World,
    New York.

   Another superb monograph from R. G.
   Wasson about the oldest and most
   widely-used hallucinogenic mushroom--
   fly agaric, Amanita muscaria. The Aryans,
   who populated the Indus valley 3500 years
   ago, are said to have used it in religio-
   magical rituals, and deified it in the
   thousand hymns of the Rig Veda.

(II:5) 225

Wasson, V. P., and R. G. Wasson. 1957.
Mushrooms, Russia and history.
Pantheon Books, New York. 2 vols.

A definitive work on fly agaric and
the other hallucinogens of importance
in northern Asia and Europe. Widely
acclaimed by ethnopharmacologists.

---

c: Biochemical and clinical
research with psychedelics

---

(II:5) 226

Aghajanian, A. K., W. E. Foote, and M. H.
Sheard. 1968. Lysergic acid diethylamide:
sensitive neuronal units in the midbrain
raphe. Science 161:706-708.

In an attempt to explain the operation of
LSD in brain chemistry, the authors injected the hallucinogen into areas of the
rat brain rich in neurons containing
serotonin, and found an irreversible ces-
sation of spontaneous nervous activity.
LSD probably serves as a serotonin anta-
gonist.

---

(II:5) 227

Antun, F., J. R. Smythies, F. Benington,
R. D. Moun, C. F. Barfknecht, and D. E.
Nichols. 1971. Native fluorescence and
hallucinogenic potency of some amphetamines. Experientia. 27(1):62-64.

The native fluorescence of a molecule
is a complex function of its electronic
reactivity, and the authors therefore
measured the fluorescence of a variety
of methoxylated amphetamines to see if
there was any correlation with hallucinogenic potency. The results indicate a
strong positive correlation, since the
least biologically active hallucinogenic
amphetamines in general showed proportion-
ately less fluorescence than the more active

ones. These experimental observations further suggest the feasibility of predicting a drug's biological activity on the basis of its electronic reactivity.

(II:5) 228

Auerbach, R., and J. A. Rugowski. 1967. Lysergic acid diethylamide: effect on embryos. Science 157:1325-1326.

Employing standard experimental procedures, the authors found that injection of LSD into 66 mice of different strains, early in pregnancy, causes a 57% incidence of gross abnormality in embryos. But the authors also note in their introduction that "a variety of agents, such as x-irradiation, viruses, drugs, vitamins, hormones and hypoxia (oxygen deficiency) are potent inducers of developmental malformations when administered to pregnant mice."

(II:5) 229

Axelrod, J., R. O. Brady, B. Witkop, and E. V. Evarts. 1957. The distribution and metabolism of lysergic acid diethylamide. Ann. N.Y. Acad. Sci. 66: 435-444.

A paper discussing the fate of the hallucinogen in the body: where it is accumulated, and how it is broken down. Dr. Axelrod has a Nobel Prize for his work on the metabolic fate of psychoactive drugs.

(II:5) 230

Bender, L., and D. V. Sivasankar. 1968. Chromosome damage not found in leukocytes of children treated with LSD-25. Science 159:749.

The authors investigated the number of chromosome breakages in white blood cells of seven schizophrenic children who had been under therapy with chemically-pure LSD-25. They observed breakages of less than 2% both in LSD-treated children and in 20 children who had not been exposed to the hallucinogen.

(II:5) 231

Budini, R., and A. Marinangeli. 1970. Interactions between some psychodrugs and flavins. Naturforsch. 25(b):505-509.

An ingenious paper. The authors find that amphetamines, LSD, and mescaline can act as electron donors to flavins, which are essential components of the body's biochemical systems concerned with energy production. Presumably the drugs interrupt the normal pathways of energy inside cells, though this remains to be authenticated.

(II:5) 232

Chothia, C., and P. Pauling. 1969. On the conformation of hallucinogenic molecules and their correlation. Proc. Nat. Acad. Sci. 63:1063-1070.

On structure and function. A technical review article providing useful references for additional reading.

(II:5) 233

Datta, R. K., and J. J. Ghosh. 1970.
  Mescaline-induced changes of brain-cortex
  ribosomes. Biochem. J. 117:961-968.

  During the action of mescaline on goat
  brain slices, the ribosomes in cells of
  this tissue became fragile and actually
  fell apart more readily than those of
  untreated preparations. Ribosomes are
  protein synthesizing structures and have
  an essential function in the process of
  memory consolidation.

(II:5) 234

Dishotsky, N. I., W. D. Longham, R. E.
  Mogar, and W. R. Lipscomb. 1971.
  LSD and genetic damage. Science 172:
  431-440.

  In this unprecedented review article the
  authors assess the findings of 68 indepen-
  dent studies conducted over the last four
  years, which have addressed themselves to
  the issue of chromosome damage caused by
  LSD. "We believe that pure LSD," they
  conclude, "ingested in moderate doses
  does not damage chromosomes in vivo,
  does not cause detectable genetic damage,
  and is not a teratogen or a carcinogen in
  man." 93 references are cited.

(II:5) 235

Evarts, E. V. 1957. A review of the neuro-
  physiological effects of lysergic acid
  diethylamide (LSD) and other psychotomimetic agents. Ann. N.Y. Acad. Sci. 66:
  479-495.

  An instructive review, even though certain information is now outdated. It
  discusses the disruption by LSD of the
  normal electrical patterns of the brain.

(II:5) 236

Fabing, H. D. 1951. New blocking agent against the development of LSD psychoses. Science 121:208.

These early investigations report the use of Meratran and a related compound as blocking agents against the model psychoses produced by LSD in humans. The gamma-isomer of Meratran is also reported to prevent or diminish central stimulation induced in the mouse by amphetamine, morphine and cocaine.

(II:5) 237

Foote, W. E., M. H. Sheard, and G. K. Aghajamian. 1969. Comparison of effects of LSD and amphetamine on midbrain raphe units. Nature 222:567-569.

Certain cells in the brain were found to respond both to LSD and amphetamine with the same electrical activity patterns. In other regions of the brain adjacent to that tested first, cells were found to respond with different electrical patterns. The authors conclude that, in some cases, LSD and amphetamine compete for the same receptors and that in other cases they do not. Although such a conclusion is ambiguous, it does illustrate the paradoxes which researchers in the field must deal with.

(II:5) 238

Friedhoff, A. J., J. W. Schweitzer, and J. Miller. 1972. Biosynthesis of mescaline and N-acetylmescaline by mammalian liver. Nature 237:454-455.

This provocative research report provides a valuable new piece of information to all interested in speculating on the chemistry of the mind. The authors have demonstrated that molecules of a known psychedelic can be biosynthesized by mistake out of chemicals already present within the mammalian body. Although the authors wisely refrain from extrapolation, their work offers yet another plausible argument in favor of the proposition that mental disorders are caused by the peculiar changes in body chemistry which cause the production of "internal" psychedelics.

(II:5) 239

Geber, W. F. 1967. Congenital malformations induced by mescaline, lysergic acid diethylamide, and bromolysergic acid in the hamster. Science 158:265-266.

Single doses of the drugs were injected into pregnant female hamsters. The unborn were subsequently found to have malformations of the brain, spinal cord, and liver, together with excessive water in the body cavity and local hemmorhages. The interesting detail of this research is that bromolysergic acid, an almost inactive LSD analogue, produced the same congenital malformations as did the fully active hallucinogen.

(II:5) 240

Giarman, N. J., and D. X. Freedman. 1965. Biochemical aspects of the action of psychotomimetic drugs. Pharmacol. Rev. 17:1-26.

A well-organized review covering the existing literature since the early thirties. A guide to many of the first scientific investigations in the field.

(II:5) 241

Gloye, E. E., and R. J. Marcus. 1970. Drug effect prediction by computer. Science 69:89-91.

The authors describe a procedure that provides automated computerized searches for patterns among the effects of drugs on the behavioral, biochemical, and physiological systems of living organisms. The computer program is expected to bring to the surface novel relationships that heretofore have been buried in medical literature.

(II:5) 242

Green, W. J. 1969. LSD and the sleep-dream cycle. Exp. Med. Surg. 27:138-144.

Experimental evidence indicates that LSD causes an increase in dream time both during and immediately after an experience with the drug.

(II:5) 243

Halaz, M. F., J. Formanek, and A. S. Marrazzi. 1969. Hallucinogen-tranquilizer interaction; its nature. Science 164:569-571.

A study of the competition between hallucinogens (STP, LSD) and tranquilizers (chlorpromazine), this paper demonstrates that a tranquilizer acts as a weak psychotomimetic protecting against a stronger one by substituting for it at the target site in the nervous system. In sufficiently large doses, the tranquilizer enhances, or, in some cases, actually produces the effect it was intended to correct.

(II:5) 244

Hofmann, A. 1959. Psychotomimetic drugs: chemical and pharmacological aspects. Acta. Physiol. Pharmacol. Neerl. 8: 240-258.

Hofmann describes the events on the afternoon of April 16, 1943 when he discovered the hallucinogenic properties of LSD while performing an experiment having to do with its synthesis. Of historical interest as an extract from a scientist's notebook.

(II:5) 245

Hollister, L. E., and A. M. Hartman. 1962. Mescaline, LSD and psilocybin: comparison of clinical syndromes, effects on color perception and biochemical measures. Comp. Psychiat. 3:235-241.

A succinct catalogue of fundamental data dealing particularly with the visual effects of the hallucinogens.

(II:5) 246

Irwin, S., and J. Egozcue. 1967. Chromosomal abnormalities in leukocytes from LSD-25 users. Science 157:313-314.

Among the first in a long series of such studies, this report describes the increase in chromosomal breakage in six out of eight volunteers who had taken LSD of their own volition before taking part in the experiment, compared with volunteers who had never taken the drug, and among whom the ratio of such breakage was only 1:9. Note that, as in most research of this type, the sample is small, and the dose as well as the purity of LSD ingested by the users is not known.

(II:5) 247

Judd, L. L., W. W. Brandkamp, and W. H. McGlothlin. 1970. Comparison of the chromosomal patterns obtained from groups of continued users, former users, and non-users of LSD-25. Amer. J. Psychiat. 12(b): 626-635.

After conducting chromosome analysis in nine heavy LSD-users who have continued use, in eight heavy users who have discontinued use, and in eight drug-free controls, the authors found no significant differences in chromosome breakage rates among any of the three groups.

(II:5) 248

Kang, S., and J. P. Green. 1970. Correlation between activity and electronic state of hallucinogenic amphetamines. Nature 226:645.

The conclusions of Snyder and Merril (Ref. #260) are confirmed in this research report.

(II:5) 249

Key, G. J. 1965. Effect of lysergic acid
diethylamide on potentials evoked in
the specific sensory pathways. Brit.
Med. Bull. 21:30-34.

Experiments on the auditory sense of
cats reported here, demonstrate that
LSD does not affect the sound-receiving
mechanism of the ear in any way. Rather,
it induces changes in processes by which
new sensory information is transformed
enroute to the auditory cortex of the
brain.

(II:5) 250

Kornetsky, C. 1970. Psychoactive drugs in the
immature organism. Psychopharmacologia.
17:105-136.

A survey of prenatal and postnatal drug
effects, emphasizing physiological and
behavioral disorders.

(II:5) 251

Multiple authors. 1968. Review section on LSD,
STP and marihuana. Amer. J. Psychiat. 125:
341-391.

In eight research papers, the following topics
are discussed by noted investigators: chronic
use of LSD by "acidheads", a statistical survey
of adverse reactions to LSD in Los Angeles
County, the effects of STP and DOET on normal
subjects, hippies and the "green rebellion",
the marihuana problem (an overview), experimental studies on marihuana, spontaneous
recurrence of the marihuana effect, and
motivation for marihuana use: a correlate
for adverse reaction. In several of the pieces,
authors compare the effects of LSD, STP and
marihuana. The overall tone of this publication
is conservative and cautious.

(II:5) 252

Rinaldi, F., and H. E. Himwich. 1955. The cerebral electrographic changes induced by LSD and mescaline are corrected by Frenquel. J. Ner. Ment. Dis. 122:424-432.

The disruption of normal electrical rhythms in the brain by a psychedelic is reversed by oral doses of the antihallucinatory drug under study. Frenquel is a trade name for azacyclonol. The drug is also used as an anti-confusion agent.

(II:5) 253

Rosenthal, S N. 1964. Persistent hallucinosis following repeated administration of hallucinogenic drugs. Amer. J. Psychiat. 121: 238-243.

Describes one of the major hazards of chronic hallucinogen use and lends support to the possibility that these chemicals may cause certain types of irreversible brain damage.

(II:5) 254

Serafetinides, H. 1965. The significance of the temporal lobes and of hemispheric dominance in the production of the LSD-25 symptomatology in man: a study of epileptic patients before and after temporal lobectomy. Neuropsychologia. 3:69-79.

Experimentation involving psychedelics and surgery on humans is rare because of justifiable ethical obstacles to this type of research, but it is occasionally done with astounding results. In this study, the author administered LSD-25 to twenty-three epileptic patients prior to the surgical removal of either their left or right temporal lobes as part of treatment for intractable epilepsy. After a series of postoperative tests, Serafetinides concluded that the perception of an LSD experience is localized almost exclusively in the right temporal lobe of the brain rather than in the left, suggesting an asymmetrical organization of the brain's regions.

(II:5) 255

Silverman, J. 1971. Research with psychedelics. Arch. Gen. Psychiat. 25:498-510.

This essay is concerned with an evaluation of the effects of psychedelic drugs, particularly LSD, on sensory function. The overriding conclusion to be drawn is that psychedelics enhance sensory experiences by stimulating specific sensory pathways in the brain. 106 recent publications on various aspects of laboratory and clinical research with psychedelic drugs is reviewed on the basis of this formulation.

(II:5) 256

Smythies, J. R., and F. Antun. 1969. Binding of tryptamine and allied compounds to nucleic acids. Nature 223:1061-1062.

The authors demonstrate that hallucinogenic tryptamines like dimethyltryptamine, ibogaine, psilocybin and their structural relative, LSD, can be bound by DNA. Through chemical association the hallucinogens may affect the reading-out of genetic information. This phenomenon has not been demonstrated in intact living systems.

(II:5) 257

Smythies, J. R. The chemical nature of the receptor site. A study in the stereochemistry of synaptic mechanisms. 1970. Int. Rev. Neurobiol. 13:181-221. Academic Press, New York.

Hallucinogens are considered to be competitive inhibitors at the site of action of serotonin. In certain cases, this inhibition is non-competitive and irreversible. The authors have assembled information lending support to each hypothesis in this up-to-date review article.

(II:5) 258

Smythies, J. R., R. J. Bradley, U. S. Johnston, F. Bennington, R. D. Morin, and L. C. Clark. 1967. Structure-activity relationship studies on mescaline. III. The influence of the methoxy groups. Psychopharmacologia 10:379-387.

Minor changes in the mescaline molecule results in considerable aberrations of the hallucinogen's biological activity. Also numerous details regarding the synthesis of mescaline and its analogues.

(II:5) 259

Snyder, S. H., and E. Richelson. 1968. Psychedelic drugs: steric factors that predict psychotropic activity. Proc. Nat. Acad. Sci. 60:206-213.

This report deals with a wide range of molecules, attempting to relate the chemical structure of psychedelic drugs to their biological and behavioral functions. An important inference to be drawn from this article is that subtle changes in molecular structure may cause pronounced changes in overall function.

(II:5) 260

Snyder, S. H., and C. R. Merril. 1965. A relationship between the hallucinogenic activity of drugs and their electronic configuration. Proc. Nat. Acad. Sci. 54:258-266.

Molecular orbital calculations have been made for a variety of hallucinogenic and non-hallucinogenic analogs of mescaline, amphetamine, tryptamine and LSD. Snyder and Merril report a close relationship between the ability to donate electrons, which depends on low molecular orbital energies, and the hallucinogenic potency of drugs. On the basis of this correlation they also predict the structure of compounds that might be more potent as hallucinogens than presently available drugs.

(II:5) 261

Stockings, G. T. 1940. Clinical study of the mescaline psychosis with special reference to the mechanisms of the genesis of schizophrenia and other psychotic states. J. Mental Sci. 86: 29-47.

The author's thesis earned a bronze medal from the Royal Medico-psychological Association and was an early catalyst for increased scientific interest in the study of drug-induced "model psychoses".

(II:5) 262

Wagner, T. E. 1969. In vitro interaction of LSD with purified calf thymus DNA. Nature 222:1170-1172.

Confirmation of observations recorded by Yielding and Sterglanz (Ref. #264).

(II:5) 263

West, L. J., C. M. Pierce, and W. D. Thomas. 1962. Lysergic acid diethylamide: its effects on a male Asiatic elephant. Science 138:1100-1103.

A classic piece of the kind of mindless research which results when scientists or clinicians hasten to publish in a trendy field. At the time of this paper LSD had just been shown to produce in humans marked mental disturbances "similar to the naturally occurring psychoses and reactions of delirium." Since bull elephants are known to suffer from a syndrome similar to psychosis called "musth"--the male equivalent of going into heat--the authors decided to try LSD on Tusko, a placid male elephant in the Oklahoma City zoo. According to the theory under investigation, the drug should have made Tusko "run berserk for a period of two weeks" as if in musth. Instead, he unceremoniously died one hour and forty minutes after the LSD had been injected.

(II:5) 264

Yielding, K. L., and H. Sterglanz. 1968.
Lysergic acid diethylamide (LSD) binding
to deoxyribonucleic acid (DNA). Proc.
Soc. Exp. Biol. Med. 128: 1096-1098.

LSD is shown to attach itself to DNA
under certain laboratory conditions.
These experiments may be interpreted
as providing a physical basis for the
hallucinogen's mutagenic effects.

Section 6:  Marihuana

    a.  Social and legal aspects
of marihuana use

(II:6) 265

Advisory Committee on Drug Dependence. 1968.
Cannabis. Her Majesty's Stationery Office,
London.

A report on the use of marihuana in
the United Kingdom, with conclusions
and recommendations. A 23-page bibliographic review of the international
clinical literature is included.

(II:6) 266

Andrews, G., and S. Vinkenoog, eds. 1967.
The book of grass, an anthology on
Indian hemp. Grove Press, New York.

A collection of brief excerpts from
the ancient and contemporary history
of marihuana. In some cases, passages
are quoted out of context, but the
anthology is excellent if only as a
sourcebook for future reference.

(II:6) 267

Bialos, D. S. 1970. Adverse marihuana
    reactions: a critical examination
    of the literature with selected
    case material. Amer. J. Psychiat.
    127:819-823.

   After considering the literature and reviewing clinical material, the author takes
   issue with the term "adverse marihuana reaction," asserting that its meaning is ambiguous when applied to describe any reactions
   to marihuana that are psychotomimetic or
   anxiety provoking or that interfere with
   functioning. "Clearly we need to know more
   about the properties of marihuana," he argues,
   "more about the personality of the people,
   and a detailed description of the setting
   before, during, and after drug use before
   we can attach value judgements to its use."

(II:6) 268

Bloomquist, E. R. 1968. Marihuana.
    Glencoe Press, Beverly Hills.

   A comprehensive study ranging from
   classical antiquity to the modern drug
   experience, presenting an objective review of reasons for marihuana usage. Dr.
   Bloomquist's personal bias is against
   the endorsement of marihuana, and his
   arguments are often cited by conservative
   clinicians for that reason.

(II:6) 269

Carstairs, G. M. 1954. Daru and Bhang: cultural
    factors in the choice of intoxicant. Quart.
    J. Stud. Alc. 15:228.

   Carstairs studied the cultural use of
   alcohol (Daru) and cannabis (Bhang) in
   northern India; concluding that the Rayputs
   prefer alcohol, and the Brahmins prefer
   marihuana. These findings are treated in
   terms of the value systems of each caste.

(II:6) 270

Chopra, R. N. 1958. Indigenous drugs of India. O. N. Duhr & Sons Private, Ltd, Calcutta.

A thorough ethnobotanical study, mostly concentrating on opium and hemp addiction.

(II:6) 271

Gamage, J. R., and E. L. Zerkin, 1969. A comprehensive guide to the English-language literature on cannabis (marihuana). STASH Bibliographic Series I. xii. STASH, Beloit.

Author and subject indices through early 1969.

(II:6) 272

Goode, E., ed. 1969. Marihuana. Atherton Press, New York.

A compendium of essays dealing with sociological and legal issues surrounding the use of marihuana. A balanced selection of opinions in succinct, well-organized prose.

(II:6) 273

Grinspoon, L. 1969. Marihuana. Sci. Am. 221: 17-25.

"There is considerable evidence that the drug is a comparatively mild intoxicant. Its current notoriety raises interesting questions about the motivation of those who use it and those who seek to punish them." Grinspoon's point is presented objectively, but he appears to be decidedly pro-marihuana.

(II:6) 274

Grinspoon, L. 1971. Marihuana reconsidered. Harvard University Press, Cambridge, Mass.

An extension of the ideas put forward in Dr. Grinspoon's *Scientific American* article. *Marihuana Reconsidered* (in hard cover and paperback) is one of the more highly regarded definitive monographs in the psychological, physiological, and social effects of marihuana in America.

(I:6) 275

Hollister, L. E. 1971. Marihuana and man: three years later. Science 172:21-29.

Dr. Hollister contends that marihuana may be unique among drugs and that the mechanisms by which it alters mental functions are not likely to be answered in man, nor even answered soon by animal studies.

(II:6) 276

Kaplan, J. 1969. Marihuana. Report of the Indian Hemp Drug Commission, 1893-94. Thomas Jefferson Publishing Company, Silver Spring.

In the last four years there has been a proliferation of writings on marihuana, and as Prof. Kaplan notes in the introduction, "those who repeat history are condemned to ignore it." Most of what is being said now was said seventy years ago, an assertion confirmed by the *Report of the Indian Hemp Drug Commission*. This 450-page document gives an insight into the whole panorama of the effect of marihuana on a culture.

(II:6) 277

Kaplan, J. 1970. Marihuana--the new prohibition. The World Publishing Company, New York.

An interesting and very well researched summary and analysis of current studies concerning the medical, social, psychiatric, and legal effects of marihuana usage, and a persuasive discussion of the possible legalization of marihuana on a "licensing model" of control. The author is a Professor of Law at Stanford University, and Fellow of the Institute for the Study of Drug Dependence in London.

(II:6) 278

Kaufman, J., J.R. Allen, and L. J. West. 1969. Runaways, hippies and marihuana. Amer. J. Psychiat. 126:717-720.

In a report based on statistics compiled in the summer of 1967 in Haight-Ashbury, the authors conclude that runaways who used the district as a refuge from society or home did not exhibit delinquent characteristics, although drugs, especially marihuana, played a complex and definable role in their behavior. The article seems to suggest that "further attempts should be directed not to the question, 'why don't they stop using drugs?', but 'can we offer them viable alternatives to drugs?'"

(II:6) 279

King, F. W. 1970. User and non-users of marihuana: some attitudinal and behavioral correlatives. J. Amer Coll. Health Assoc. 18:213-217.

A discussion of statistics compiled at Dartmouth College. In the conclusion, King notes that "neither knowing someone who has used marihuana nor actually having the opportunity to try marihuana automatically seduces all students into using the drug."

(II:6) 280

Mayor's Committee on Marihuana. 1944. The Marihuana problem in the city of New York. Jacques Cattell Press, Lancaster, Pa.

Mayor La Guardia's report is a fundamental document invariably cited by any commentator on marihuana use and abuse. More than twenty-five years ago, the Mayor's Committee advocated reform of laws placing marihuana in the same category as heroin, and stipulating similar punishment for infractions. The committee also noted that marihuana use did not necessarily lead to use of narcotics and other drugs.

(II:6) 281

McGlothlin, W., K. Jamison, and S. Rosenblatt. 1970. Marihuana and the use of other drugs. Nature 228:1227-1229.

During Operation Intercept, the suppy of marihuana in 1969 dwindled to the point that accustomed users sought harder drugs as a substitute. The authors cite statistical evidence in support of this proposition and question the validity of social policies directed at controlling one drug which leads to increased use of competing-- and perhaps more dangerous intoxicants.

(II:6) 282

Orcutt, J. D. 1972. Toward a sociological theory of drug effects: a comparison of marihuana and alcohol. Sociol. Soc. Res. 56:242-253.

An attempt to reach a social definition of the effects of the "new social drug" marihuana in comparison to the effects of the "old social drug," alcohol. The author presents a scheme by which the two drugs can be conceptually distinguished as functions of three sociological determinants which he calls "normative content," "normative clarity," and "situational context."

(II:6) 283

Rand, M. E., W. Goaf, and C. Thurlow. 1970.
    Alcohol or marihuana. A follow-up
    survey at Ithaca College. J. Amer.
    Coll. Health Assoc. 18:366-367.

   The original study was conducted in 1967
   and indicated that 29% of the males and
   18% of the females had used marihuana.
   More recent data indicates that "among
   college students, the illegal use of
   psychotomimetic drugs is a majority
   experience."

(II:6) 284

Rosevear, J. 1967. Pot, a handbook of
    marihuana. University Books, New
    Hyde Park, New York.

   Mostly sociological in coverage, this short
   book presents interdisciplinary criticism
   on the uses and abuses of the intoxicant.
   Recommended only for historical reasons
   since it has been dated by more recent
   studies of the subject.

(II:6) 285

Select Committee on Crime. 1970. Marihuana,
    first report. U. S. Government Print-
    ing Office, Washington, D. C.

   A report to the House of Representatives
   including transcripts of testimony on drug
   abuse, law enforcement, and marihuana
   penalties. The members of the Select
   Committee concluded that the marihuana
   problems will not be solved by proponents
   of the extreme sides of the issue--not
   by those who contend that "drug use is a
   symptom of the degeneracy of our youth
   and who wildly proclaim that such depravity should be 'stamped out', "nor by
   those who advocate the use and extol the
   virtues of psychedelic compounds." In
   addition, the committee calls for revision

of the laws controlling marihuana "to make the penalties relating to violations rational and then to bring about uniform and even enforcement of laws."

(II:6) 286

Simmons, J. L. 1967. Marihuana. Myths and realities. Brandon House, Hollywood.

A hard-hitting, short book intended to popularize approaches to a rational view of marihuana. The information is clearly presented and easy to follow. Recommended for historical reasons since it was one of the first popular primers on fact and opinion about the drug's use in a social setting.

(II:6) 287

Solomon, D. 1960. The marihuana papers. Bobbs-Merrill Company, Indianapolis.

A thorough review of the older marihuana literature, touching on science, history, sociology, culture and imagination. Highly recommended by reviewers for the scope and depth of its coverage, Solomon's collection is a recognized classic, although the vigorous endorsement of marihuana is considered unwarranted by social critics.

(II:6) 288

Smith, D. E., ed. 1970. The new social drug. Prentice-Hall, Englewood Cliffs, N. J.

A sophisticated anthology of cultural, medical, and legal perspectives concerning the use of marihuana in the contemporary social setting. Essays by distinguished contributors interpret marihuana use as a middle-class phenomenon gaining wide acceptance despite legal deterrents, and possible health hazards. The editor practices and teaches in San Francisco, edits The Journal of New Drugs and has gained recognition as an expert on the Haight-Ashbury subculture.

(II:6) 289

Tart, G. T. 1970. Marihuana intoxication: common experiences. Nature 226:701-704.

    The author presents a summary of the chief experimental effects of marihuana which were elucidated with the help of a detailed questionnaire given to seasoned marihuana users. The data suggests that marihuana's actions upon perception, thought processing, and interpersonal relationships are almost entirely beneficial. This is one of the less well known but valuable studies on the subject.

(II:6) 290

Walton, R. P. 1938. Marihuana: America's new drug problem. J. P. Lippincott Company, Philadelphia.

    Important as an extensive review of the older literature on marihuana, particularly of the period around the turn of the century.

    b: Biochemical and clinical research on marihuana

(II:6) 291

Clark, L. D., R. Hughes, and E. N. Nakashima. 1970. Behavioral effects of marihuana. Arch. Gen. Psychiat. 23:193-203.

    Evidence is presented suggesting that marihuana has significant effects on complex reaction time, recent memory, recall, and comprehension of written information. It should be noted that in this series of experiments, an extract of bulk marihuana was prepared and administered orally: the effects of the drug administered under these conditions are known to differ from those elicited when the drug is smoked.

(II:6) 292

Goode, E. 1969. Multiple drug use among marihuana smokers. Soc. Prob. 17:48-64.

Data from 204 interviews permits the following conclusions: use of strong drugs, primarily the psychedelics, increases with increased marihuana use, but infrequent marihuana use does not inevitably lead to its frequent use.

(II:6) 293

Holtzman, D., R. A. Lovell, J. H. Jaffe, and D. X. Freedman. 1969. 1- 9-tetrahydrocannabinol: neurochemical and behavioral effects in the mouse. Science 163:1464-1467.

Information of value only for comparative studies. A series of routine but carefully executed experiments leads the authors to conclude that the characteristic change in the chemistry of brain amines produced by the active ingredient of marihuana does not correspond to those observed with other drugs, including barbiturates and LSD.

(II:6) 294

Keup, W. 1970. Psychotic symptoms due to cannabis abuse. Dis. Nerv. Syst. 31:119-126.

In a survey of newly-admitted mental patients over a twelve-month period, the author reports that "in 0.9 per thousand of all admissions was cannabis found to be the direct cause of hospitalization. In an additional 1.9 per thousand it was a contributory factor." The article also offers a catalogue of psychiatric consequences of cannabis abuse, including acute intoxication, echo-reactions, psychoses, and lasting mental decline and character changes (mostly reported from Eastern countries).

(II:6) 295

Kudrin, A. N., and O. N. Davydova. An agent for the elimination of hashish action in dogs. Farmakol. Toksikol. 31:549.

The Russian researchers report that they can counteract cannabis intoxication by injecting a nitropropiophenone drug into test animals either before or after exposure to the intoxicant. The new drug is considered to be of potential use as an antidote.

(II:6) 296

Lemberg, L., S. D. Silberstein, J. Axelrod, and I. Kopin, 1970. Marihuana: studies on the disposition and metabolism of delta-9-tetrahydrocannabinol in man. Science 170:1320-1322.

A team of researchers from the National Institute of Mental Health report in this publication that delta-9-tetrahydrocannabinol (THC) administered intravenously to three volunteers persists in their blood stream for more than three days and that breakdown products linger for more than eight days. Although these findings received wide coverage in the news media shortly after their publication, their signifi-

cance to the overall study of marihuana use remains in question. Few, if any, marihuana advocates obtain highs by taking pot or its major active component, THC, intravenously. Rather, marihuana is usually smoked so that a whole series of combustion products are taken into the body. It is the disposition and metabolism of these chemicals that should be studied.

(II:6) 297

McIsaac, W. M., G. E. Fritchie, J. E. Idapaan-Heikkita, B. T. Ho, and L. F. Anglert. 1971. Distribution of marihuana in monkey brain and concommitant behavioral effects. Nature 230:593-594.

Monkeys were injected with radioactively labelled tetrahydrocannabinol (THC) and then sacrificed after suitable intervals. Extremely high concentrations of THC were found in the frontal cortex and the hippocampus, two areas of the brain which regulate event perception. This finding correlates well with behavioral observations, since one of the chief effects of marihuana is distortion of time perception. The researchers also observed that practically

no radioactive THC accumulated in the hypothalamus, a region that controls aggressiveness. There exists thus an obvious difference between THC and STP, since the hallucinogenic amphetamine STP does accumulate in the hypothalamus where it is presumed to trigger antisocial and aggressive behavior.

(II:6) 298

Mechoulam, R. 1970. Marihuana chemistry. Science 168:1159-1166.

A review of recent advances, the most controversial of which are treated in the author's critical evaluation of known syntheses for tetrahydrocannabinol, the active ingredient in marihuana.

(II:6) 299

Melges, F. T., J. R. Tinklenberg, L. F. Hollister, and H. K. Gillespie. 1970. Marihuana and temporal disintegration. Science 168:1118-1120.

High doses of marihuana extracts taken orally significantly impaired the coordination of the test subjects during a task requiring sequential adjustments toward reaching a goal. This disintegration of sequential thought processes is related to impaired immediate memory. The authors concede, however, that the 40-60 mg. doses used are "probably considerably higher than those obtained from the usual custom of smoking marihuana in social settings."

(II:6) 300

Melges, F. T., J R. Tinklenberg, L. E. Hollister, and H. K. Gillespie. 1970. Temporal disintegration and depersonalization during marihuana intoxication. Arch. Gen. Psychiat. 23:204-210.

As in the previous study, the drug was administered orally. The overall findings indicate that ingestion of marihuana causes euphoria and fragmentation of temporal experience.

(II:6) 301

National Library of Medicine Literature Searches. 1969. Cannabis toxicology. Dept. of Health, Education and Welfare, U.S. Government Printing Office, Washington, D.C.

A bibliography covering 55 references from January 1964 to August 1968.

(II:6) 302

National Library of Medicine Literature
  Searches. 1972. Cannabis toxicology.
  Dep. of Health, Education and Welfare,
  U.S. Government Printing Office,
  Washington, D.C.

This bibliography, consisting of
355 citations to literature on the
adverse effects of marihuana, covers
the period from September 1968 to
July 1971.

(II:6) 303

Neumeyer, J. L., and R. A. Shagowry. 1971.
  Chemistry and pharmacology of marihuana.
  J. Pharmaceut. Sci. 60:1433-1458.

A more extensive and technical review of
the subject than those already cited. It
is intended for readers with a first-hand
knowledge of organic chemistry. The authors
cite 211 publications.

Section 7: Inhalants

(II:7) 304

Weil, A. T., N. E. Zinberg, and J. M. Nelsen.
  1968. Clinical and psychological effects
  of marihuana in man. Science 162:1234-1242.

The authors have produced clarifications
of several nagging misconceptions about
marihuana, especially regarding users'
heart rate, metabolism, muscular coordination, and task performance. In addition,
this report is a cornerstone to the
methodology by which the effects of similar
"mild intoxicants" can be evaluated as im-
partially as possible.

(II:7) 305

Bearg, R. D. 1971. Centrilobular hepatic
   necrosis and acute renal failure in
   "solvent sniffers". Ann. Intern. Med.
   73:713-720.

   This research report emphasizes the devastating consequences of glue sniffing. The volatile chemicals often inhaled by children may cause severe liver and kidney malfunctions.

(II:7) 306

Barker, G. H., and W. T. Adams. 1963. Glue
   sniffers. Sociol. Soc. Res. 47:298-310.

   A study of the personality traits, motivations and habits of glue sniffers. The word "glue" here covers a wide variety of volatile inhalants commonly used by children and teenagers.

(II:7) 307

Browning, E. 1963. Toxic Solvents.
   Chemical Publications Company,
   New York.

   A definitive handbook on the chemical properties of paint thinners, cleaning fluids, gasoline, and industrial solvents. Many of these are used by inhalation to produce intoxication or euphoria, but often can lead to sudden death due to effects on the heart. They also can produce extensive damage to kidney, liver, and bone marrow.

(II:7) 308

Daly, C. D., and R. White. 1930. Psychic
   reactions to olfactory stimuli.
   Brit. J. Med. Psychol. 10:70-87.

   An analysis of the "nature" of the pleasure obtained from sniffing various chemical fumes. This is one of the few studies on the psychological effects of adolescent activities such as glue sniffing.

(II:7) 309

Fitzherbert, J. 1959. Scent and sexual object. Brit. J. Med. Psychol. 32:206-209.

The phenomenon of glue sniffing is illustrated here as part of a coping mechanism which permits the user to face certain realities about himself during a period of adolescent sexual adjustment.

(II:7) 310

Kupperstein, L. R., and R. M. Sussman. 1968. A bibliography on the inhalation of glue fumes and other toxic vapors--a substance abuse practice among adolescents. Int. J. Addict. 3:177-198.

A bibliographic survey of literature on the intoxicating and euphoriating effects of nitrous oxide, ethyl ether, glue and other volatile compounds.

(II:7) 311

Press, E., and A. K. Done. 1967. Solvent sniffing. Ped. 29:451-461;611-622.

A compilation of medical information. The authors review the physiological consequences of "cheap kicks" produced by exposure to the highly volatile vapors of lacquers, enamels, paint thinners, paint and varnish removers, brake and lighter fluids, and plastic cements.

(II:7) 312

Reinhardt, C. F. 1971. Cardiac arrhythmias and aerosol "sniffing". Arch. Environ. Health. 22:265-279.

Various kinds of heart trouble are cited as a consequence of glue sniffing.

Section 8: Chemical Indentification and Clinical Diagnosis of Psychoactive Drugs

(II:8) 313

Wayne, G. G., and A. A. Clinco. 1959. Psychoanalytic observations on olfaction with special reference to olfactory dreams. Psychoanalysis Psychoanal. Rev. 46(4):64-79.

This classic paper shows how certain highly pleasant dream experiences are associated with certain smells. Its import within the context of studies on drug abuse lies in the suggestion that "glue sniffers" are motivated toward their habit by association with a pleasurable dream world brought about by the "smell" of glue.

(II:8) 314

Belmann, S. W., J. W. Turczan, and T. C. Kram. 1970. Spectrophotometric forensic chemistry of hallucinogenic drugs. J. Forensic Sci. 15(2):261-286.

A thorough technical article describing the application of sensitive spectroscopic techniques used by organic chemists for the identification of hallucinogens, including LSD, mescaline, and MDA.

(II:8) 315

Cheek, F. E., S. Newell, and M. Joffe. 1970. Deceptions in the illicit drug market. Science 167:1276.

After analyzing forty-four "street" drug samples, the investigators report that "while most of the samples said to be LSD were actually LSD, none of the samples said to be mescaline, psilocybin, or THC were those substances. Four of the samples said to be mescaline were actually STP."

(II:8) 316

Davidow, B., N Li Pietri, and B. Duane. 1968.
A thin layer chromatographic screening procedure for detecting drug abuse. Amer. J. Clin. Pathol. 38:714-719.

A comprehensive, short review article on this simple technique for the qualitative identification of drugs. Data is cited for 89 of the most commonly abused tranquilizers, stimulants, and narcotics, but the psychedelics and marihuana are not included.

(II:8) 317

De Gross, J. 1971. Emergency treatment of drug abuse and poison ingestion. J. Med. Times. 99:53-64.

Designed as a guide for physicians. The article concerns itself with the problem of antidote selection.

(II:8) 318

Silva, J. A. F. de, and L. d'Arconte. 1969. The use of spectrofluorometry in the analysis of drugs in biological materials. J. Forensic Sci. 14:184-204.

An exhaustive survey, valuable primarily because the authors offer summaries of the methodology currently applied in drug research for the qualitative identification and quantitative determination of minute amounts--not only of drugs but of their metabolites. In particular, the authors discuss the use of fluorescence techniques.

(II:8) 319

Dimijian, G C. 1970. Clinical evaluation of the drug users: current concepts. Texas Med. 66:42-49.

A description of major and minor symptom categories intended as a diagnostic aid for physicians and laymen. Includes recommendations regarding treatment.

(II:8) 320

Gunn, J. W., D. W. Johnson, and W. P. Butler. Clandestine drug laboratories. J. Forensic Sci. 15:51-64.

The when and how of illegal LSD, STP, DMT, DET, mescaline, psilocybin and other drug manufacture. The authors note that "the drugs produced are of unknown quality, which in itself is a danger to users."

(II:8) 321

Kaitstha, K. K. 1972. Drug abuse screening programs: detection procedures, development costs, street-sample analysis, and field tests. J. Pharmaceut. Sci. 61:655-678.

A noteworthy review covering 253 publications about the techniques used to identify all the classes of drugs in clinical and toxicological laboratories.

(II:8) 322

Keller, R. A., ed. 1972. Analysis of drugs of abuse. J. Chromatog. Sci. 10:(May)

This special issue is devoted entirely to the subject of drug analysis from a research, clinical, forensic, and law-enforcement point of view. All articles included present information in a manner that will be particularly appealing to readers with a peripheral knowledge of analytical chemistry. Another asset of this particular compilation lies in the final article titled "A bibliography of references on the analysis of drugs of abuse," which lists over 400 publications.

(II:8) 323

Lerner, M., and M. D. Katsiaficas. 1969. Analytical separations of mixtures of hallucinogenic drugs. Bull. Narcotics 21: 47-51.

> A short article describing two of the most commonly used techniques for the identification of hallucinogens. Experimental results of gas liquid chromatography and thin-layer chromatography are reported for LSD, mescaline, psilocybin, and related compounds.

(II:8) 324

Niyogi, S. K. 1970. Methods of separation of drugs from biological materials. J Forensic Med. 17:72-95.

> On the extraction and characterization of representative tranquilizers and narcotics from human blood, urine, and postmortem viscerae. The author offers a critique of the methodology and 169 references to the pertinent scientific literature.

(II:8) 325

Schwartz, M., ed. 1972. Clinical methods for drugs of abuse. Bendix Corporation, Roncerverte, West Virginia.

> A two-volume compendium of techniques for the diagnosis and chemical analysis of alcohols, barbiturates, amphetamines, and alkaloids (including opiates and hallucinogens). Unfortunately these two books are not in wide circulation, but can be obtained directly from the Bendix Corporation.

(II:8) 326

Sohn, D., and J. Simon. 1970. Narcotics detection and industry. J. Occup. Med. 12:6-9.

> A short, practical review of the methodology currently available for the routine identification of drugs and drug mixtures.

(II:8) 327

Sunshine, I., ed. 1969. Handbook of analytical toxicology. The Chemical Rubber Company, Cleveland.

This manual brings together a mass of data which has been scattered throughout the literature pertaining to the chemical identification of drugs and poisonous substances. It is also especially commendable for its time saving, though extensive, index. A new edition of this book should be available by 1973.

(II:8) 328

Taylor, R. L., J. I. Maurer, and J. R. Tinklenberg. 1970. Management of bad trips in an evolving drug scene. J. Amer. Med. Assoc. 213(3):422-425.

Operating under the well-chosen premise that rational therapy for "bad trips" must consider completely social, psychological, and physiological factors, the authors have set down practical guidelines for the evaluation and treatment of the "bad tripper." According to their experience in hundreds of clinical trials, the fundamental rule in the management of "bad trips" is the establishment of verbal contact with the minimum use of tranquilizers. Additional forms of treatment are also discussed.

(II:8) 329

Turk, R. F., H. I. Dharir, and R. B. Forney. 1969. A simple chemical method to identify marihuana. J. Forensic Sci. 14:389-393.

An amplification of the results reported in Ref. #330.

(II:8) 330

Turk, R. F., R. B. Forney, L. J. King, and S. Ramachandran. 1969. A method for extraction and chromatographic isolation, purification and identification of tetrahydrocannabinol and other compounds from marihuana. J. Forensic. Sci. 14: 385-389.

Together with the preceding paper, this is the best published procedure for analytical techniques in marihuana chemistry. Unfortunately, the journal is a hard one to come by.

# CHAPTER III

# Drugs in Society

## Section 1: Drugs and the Young

(III:1) 331

Anumonye, A., and J. L. McClure. 1970. Adolescent drug abuse in a north London suburb. Brit. J. Addict. 65:25-33.

Information gathered from 54 patients is analyzed in order to correlate demographic, sociological and medical histories.

(III:1) 332

Black, S., K. L. Ownes, and R. P. Wolff. 1970. Patterns of drug use: a study of 5,482 subjects. Amer. J. Psychiat. 127: 420-423.

A study based on one of the largest samples studied in current literature. 23% of the subjects interviewed were found to have tried marihuana, 7% LSD, 10% amphetamines, and 1.6% heroin. The authors report that "although initial experiences with marihuana tend to lead to continued use, marihuana usage does not lead most individuals into experimentation with heroin."

(III:1) 333

Brotmas, R., I. Silverman, and F. Suffet. 1970. Some social correlates of student drug use. Crime and Delin. 16:67-74.

A study comparing drug users and non-users from the student body of a private high school in New York City. Drug users were found to display attitudes such as opposition to war in Vietnam, occasional participation in sports, negligible church attendance, and political radicalism. The authors attribute these attitudes to underlying sociological maladjustments rather than to drug abuse.

(III:1) 334

Carey, J. J. 1968. The college drug scene. Prentice-Hall, Englewood Cliffs, N.J.

This book suffers by comparison with other offerings on the subject of drugs and the college campus; the author proposes to understand the alienation, goals and realities of "grass" and "acid" users, but fails to convey any such understanding, partially owing to the fragmentary way in which his information is presented. The book reads like a series of loosely-connected paragraphs. A sympathetic, but non-innovative presentation.

(III:1) 335

Carson, D. I., and J. M. Lewis. 1970. Factors influencing drug abuse in young people. Texas Med. 66:50-57.

Drug abuse in adolescents is attributed to a combination of cultural, familial and individual factors. Under the latter category are included loneliness, sexual conflicts, self-destructive tendencies, etc. Not an especially innovative article, but presents a useful overview.

(III:1) 336

Cohen, H. 1970. Principal conclusions from the report: "psychology, social-psychology, and sociology of illicit drug use." Brit. J. Addict. 65:39-44.

Using material deriving from a survey of 958 respondents in Holland, the author concludes that most respondents had not restricted their drug use to any one illicit drug. Statistics on LSD and marihuana are discussed from a sociological standpoint.

(III:1) 337

Cohen, M., and D. F. Klein. 1970. Drug abuse in a young psychiatric population. Amer. J. Orthopsychiat. 40:448-455.

A statistical study based on data obtained from patients of the Hillside Hospital in New York. Results indicate that "heavy drug users were more likely to be character disorders than psychotic, and were of higher intelligence than non-drug users."

(III:1) 338

Davis. F., and L. Munoz. 1968. Heads and freaks: patterns and meanings of drug abuse among hippies. J. Health Soc. Behav. 9:156-164.

This article should be consulted for historical and philosophical purposes. It contains detailed analyses of the popular terminology used during the hey-day of psychedelic drug use in California. Many of the words listed, though, have now fallen into disuse.

(III:1) 339

Drug abuse project report to the Ford Foundation. 1972. Dealing with drug abuse. Prager, New York.

A survey of nine different drug-treatment programs in New York. It covers intelligently the nature of the drug problem in urban areas and examines suggestively the disarray of drug education schemes, the sins of the pharmaceutical establishment, and the paucity of law-enforcement policies.

(III:1) 340

Gilbert, B. Drugs in sports. Sports Illustrated 30(25):64-72; 30(26):30-42; 31(1):30-35.

On the illegal use of stimulants and tranquilizers to modify athletes' performances under conditions of stress in competition.

(III:1) 341

Gitchoff, G. T. 1969. Kids, cops and kilos: a study of contemporary suburban youth. Malter-Westerfield, San Diego.

A lively account of the extent to which the counter-culture has penetrated the heretofore unpenetrable barriers of suburbia. Good for the authors' psychological analysis of suburbia's response to this intrusion.

(II:1) 342

Goethals, G. W., and S. Klos. 1970. Experiencing youth. Little, Brown and Company. Boston.

This is a book of autobiographical studies of Harvard-Radcliffe students. Included is one case study of a heavy drug user.

(III:1) 343

Goode, E. 1972. Drug use and grades in college. Nature 234:225-227.

A survey conducted during January and February of 1970 on 560 students attending Dr. Goode's truancy and delinquency classes at the State University of New York at Stoney Brook.

(III:1) 344

Greder. J. F., and D. W. Morgan. 1972.
Patterns of drug abuse and attitudes
toward treatment in a military population.
Arch. Gen. Psychiat. 26:113-117.

Data from a questionnaire survey conducted
on 747 enlisted men at Fort Lee, Virginia.
Fifty percent of these men reported that
they were drug users, although to varying
extents.

(III:1) 345

Herzog, E. 1970. Drug use among the young:
as teenagers see it. Children 17:207-212.

A statistical survey. One of the few
compilations of data on under-18 drug
users.

(III:1) 346

Imperi, L. L., H. D. Kleber, and J. S. Davie.
1968. Use of hallucinogenic drugs on campus. J. Amer. Med. Assoc. 104(12):1021-1024.

Statistics and clinical commentary
compiled roughly from 1965 to 1967.

(III:1) 347

Irgens-Jensen. O., and S. Burn-Gulbrandsen.
1971. Drugs in Norway: attitudes and
use. Int. J. Addic. 6:109-118.

An historical and statistical summary
of drug abuse in Norway since 1950.
In particular the authors examine the
long-term effects of severe penalties
imposed for minor drug offenses.

(III:1) 348

Jacobs, M. A., and A. Z. Spilken. 1971. Personality patterns associated with heavy cigarette smoking in male college students. J. Consult. Clin. Psychiat. 37:428-432.

This study reveals that many of the personality traits which characterize hard drug users also apply to inveterate smokers.

(III:1) 349

Johnson, K. G., H. Donnelly, R. Scheble, R. L. Wine, and M. Weitman. 1971. Survey of adolescent drug use. I. Sex and grade distribution. Am. J. Pub. Health 61:2418-2432.

This article presents the data from a questionnaire survey of drug use among 2,752 high school students in Portland and Multnomah County, Oregon. The survey, conducted in the spring of 1968, covered marihuana, amphetamines, inhalants, sedatives, tranquilizers, cocaine, hallucinogens, narcotics, alcohol, tobacco, headache remedies, and cold remedies. This article is particularly worthy of mention because according to the authors, "presentation of the data by sex and grade distribution discloses that more boys than girls report using each of the drugs except barbiturates, antihistamines, sedatives, tranquilizers, and headache remedies."

(III:1) 350

Johnson, K.G., H. Abbey, R. Scheble, and M. Weitman, 1972. Survey of adolescent drug use. II. social and environmental factors. Am. J. Pub. Health 62:164-166.

The second in a novel three-part series, this publication correlates drug abuse with the following 12 demographic, social or environmental characteristics: broken families, income less than $3,000, nonwhite population, aid to dependent children, adult crime, juvenile delinquency, substandard housing, housing value less than $5,000, rent less than $60 per month, renter occupancy, crowded housing, and general social climate. This analysis

shows that adolescent drug abuse is positively associated with the demographic characteristics which are usually accepted as indicators of pathogenic environment.

(III:1) 351

Loiselle, P., and P. C. Whitehead. 1971. Scaling drug use: an examination of the popular wisdom. Canad. J. Behav. Sci. 3: 347-356.

This statistical study offers compelling evidence in favor of debunking the notion that marihuana smoking is a stepping stone to heroin addiction. "Drug use," state the authors, "is not a unidimensional phenomenon." Thirty-seven references are cited.

(III:1) 352

McGlothlin, W. H., and S. Cohen. 1965. The use of hallucinogenic drugs among college students. Am. J. Psych. 122:572-574.

Useful for comparison with current surveys. The incidence of drug use appears to be decidedly lower then than at present, according to data presented here.

(III:1) 353

Mizner, G. L., J T. Barter, and P. H. Werme. 1970. Patterns of drug use among college students: a preliminary report. Amer. J. Psychiat. 127:55-64.

    A carefully-executed survey of the Denver-Boulder metropolitan area. Data on marihuana, amphetamines and LSD is presented and includes reasons for drug use, reported lifetime drug use by school, and plans for future use.

(III:1) 354

Nowlis, H. H. 1969. Drugs on the college campus. Doubleday-Anchor, Garden City, New York.

    A "concerned" review of facts and issues along the same lines as an earlier work by Young and Hixson (Ref. #367). The interpretations are of necessity inconclusive but effectively presented, and the book has been cited in several current publications.

(III:1) 355

Phillips, A. F 1967. The campus drug problem. J. Amer. Coll. Health Assoc. 16:150-160.

    A general discussion. The academic year 1967-68 marked the turning point after which drug use on the campus became "drug abuse" and consequently a "problem".

(III:1) 356

Pope, G. 1972. Voices from the drug culture. Beacon Press, Boston.

    Discusses the use by young people of certain illicit drugs as a response to the boredom and superficiality they perceive in American society. Includes many direct quotations from users.

(III:1) 357

Smart, R. G. 1971. Illicit drug use in Canada: a review of current epidemology with clues for prevention. Int. J. Addict. 6:383-405.

A re-evaluation of previous statistical studies on marihuana, LSD, and speed abuse by some segments of the Canadian population. 21 references.

(III:1) 358

Smith, B. C. 1970. Drug use on a university campus. J. Amer. Coll. Health Assoc. 18:360-365.

Current statistics from the University of Florida. The authors conclude that "not many students want to experience drugs beyond alcohol and marihuana."

(III:1) 359

Stanton, M. D. 1972. Drug use in Vietnam. Arch. Gen. Psychiat. 26:279-286.

This survey reports on the drug experience, marihuana smoking in particular, of 2,547 army personnel. The data summarized here was compiled in 1969.

(III:1) 360

Stearn, J. 1969. The seekers: drugs and the new generation. Doubleday, New York.

The sort of book parents give an oldest son on his eighteenth birthday. A noble attempt to invent catchy phrases and analogies, but a half-baked product, altogether.

(III:1) 361

Torgo, R., and P. Kaminstein. 1972. Cooptive intervention: the case of the storefront drug center. Adolescence 26:183-198.

The article evaluates the viability of a model federally sponsored storefront drug information center. The name of the center is not revealed, but it is located adjacent to the business district of a medium-size industrial city in the Northeast.

(III:1) 362

Ungerleider, J. T., and H. L. Bowen. 1969. Drug abuse and the schools. Am. J. Psychiat. 125:1691-1697.

In a sensitive appraisal of the situation, the authors assert that "preventive programs must include the development of open communication about drugs. Applying the ombudsman approach to drug problems within the schools is one effective way of achieving this." Specific details of this approach used while working with California high school students are discussed.

(III:1) 363

Walters, P., G. W. Goethals, and H. G. Pope. 1972. Drug use and life-style among 500 college undergraduates. Arch. Gen. Psychiat. 26:92-96.

In this study, conducted on seniors at Harvard University in 1969, the authors report that "no differences were found between users and non-users in relation to grades, athletics, and activities;" but significant differences were found between the two groups with regard to pre-existing self-concepts, values, and attitudes unrelated to "official" college life.

(III:1) 364

Weil, A. T. 1963. The strange case of the Harvard drug scandal. Look. 5 Nov:38-48.

An inside-Harvard view of the Leary days through the eyes of an observer noted for his shrewdness and perceptiveness. Dr. Weil has taught at Harvard and is author of several publications dealing with marihuana and other "social" drugs.

(III:1) 365

Weitman, M., R. Schele, K. G. Johnson, and H. Asbey. 1972. Survey of adolescent drug use. III. Correlations among use of drugs. Am. J. Pub. Health 62:166-170.

In this final paper of the series, the authors present statistical data which helps define the relationships between drugs of abuse. Of particular interest are the correlations between use of marihuana and the use of alcohol, tobacco, amphetamines, barbiturates, hallucinogens, and narcotics.

(III:1) 366

Wittenborn, J. R., H. Brill, J P. Smith, and S. A. Wittenborn. 1969. Drugs and youth. Proceedings of the Rutgers symposium on drug abuse. Charles C. Thomas, Springfield, Illinois.

A recent interdisciplinary report covering historical overviews, abuse of tranquilizers, stimulants, opiates, psychedelics, and cannabis alkaloids, outstanding for its concluding section, titled "Action", a sensitive appraisal of the course to be charted by government and private institutions in adjusting to the drug cult.

(III:1) 367

Young, W. R., and J. R. Hixson. 1966. LSD
    on campus. Dell, New York.

   Although the actual information presented
   here is neither unique nor especially significant compared to currently-available
   statistics, this book merits consideration
   as the reflection of a typically parental
   viewpoint: worry and amazement over the
   sociological and cultural transformations
   being undergone by people of college age.

(III:1) 368

Zinberg, N. D. 1972. Heroin use in Vietnam
    and the United States.
    Arch. Gen. Psychiat. 26:486-488.

   Dr. Zinberg offers a critique of the
   comparative data on heroin use in the
   United States and Vietnam. "Heroin use
   by American soldiers in Vietnam," he
   writes, "differs significantly from
   heroin use in the United States. Users
   in Vietnam are of many personality types
   and backgrounds and most have slight
   previous drug experience...most important,
   users are members of small heroin-taking
   groups who are disillusioned with the
   'non-war' and the Army in contrast to the
   'loner' user in the United States."

Section 2:   Drugs in the Sociology and
             Politics of the Counterculture

(III:2) 369

Agnew, D. 1959. Undercover agent--narcotics.
    McFadden-Bartell, New York.

   A short, partially autobiographical
   account of the life and times of a
   Bureau of Narcotics agent. Agnew
   pursues criminals, deplores the use
   of drugs, and ardently advocates law
   and order.

(III:2) 370

Adler, N. 1970. Kids, drugs and politics. Psychoanal. Rev. 57:432-441.

    The politics of ecstasy as seen by the somewhat skeptical analyst.

---

(III:2) 371

Barber, B. 1967. Drugs and society. Russell Sage Foundation.

    Barber is primarily concerned with the problem of education and communication and the role of the media in disseminating information about drugs. In the final chapter, he discusses aesthetic, psychic, political, ideological, aphrodisiac and therapeutical functions of drugs.

---

(III:2) 372

Bewley, T. H. 1967. Some social, psychological and environmental factors associated. Health Educ. J. 16:60-66.

    A general survey correlating the causes of the drug culture with its visible manifestations. The article deals mostly with the psychological problems of modern youth.

---

(III:2) 373

Bleibtraub, J. N. 1967. Marihuana and the new American hedonism. Psychedel. Rev. 9:72-80.

    "The link between capitalism and the Puritan ethic may be responsible for the national opposition to a benign pleasure-giving weed." After this epigraph Bleibtraub proceeds to demonstrate that hedonism will ultimately win out starting in 1970. "I think one can predict," he asserts at the end, "that both the moral and statutory opposition to marihuana smoking will slacken."

(III:2) 374

Blos, P. 1962. On adolescence. Free Press, Glencoe, Illinois.

> An excellent study on the identity problem of youth, but it is very technical work and intended for readers who are conversant with psychoanalytic theory.

(III:2) 375

Blum, J., and J. Smith. Nothing left to lose. Sanctuary, Cambridge, Mass.

> Case studies of street people based on the experiences of counselors at a Cambridge-based center, the Sanctuary. This book discusses the societal forces that lead young people to leave home, the failures of established institutions to help these young people, and the counseling techniques used by Sanctuary staff in working with them. (Second edition has been published by Beacon Press.)

(III:2) 376

Blum, R. H. et al. 1970. Society and drugs. Jossey-Bass Inc., San Francisco. 2 vol.

> An impartial collation of historical and sociological information already published in over a thousand books and articles, Blum's two volumes of essays are the closest approximation to a portable library of non-scientific literature about drugs. An invaluable guide.

(III:2) 377

Brickman, H. R. 1968. The psychedelic "hip scene": return of the death instinct. Amer. J. Psychiat. 125(6):766-772.

> The author traces the origins of the "non-violent subculture" and its non-violent ethic within the frame of reference of Freud's theory of the death instinct. The psychedelic episode and the experience of ego dissolution (dying) are seen in intimate connection--confirming the basic unity of life and death and therefore eliminating the individual's need to externalize destructiveness.

(III:2) 378

Brown, J. D., ed. 1967. The hippies.
    Time-Life Books, New York.

   A cleverly-written, subtle and percep-
   tive commentary on the hippie life style
   as it had evolved through the use of
   psychedelics in the early and middle
   sixties.

(III:2) 379

Brown, N O. 1966. Love's body.
    Random House, New York.

   A speculative account of the fate of
   the voracious ego, i.e. the twentieth-
   century seer-psychopath-revolutionary
   who wishes to merge with the whole world,
   break through into eternity, and usher
   in a new dimension of chaos. Considered
   to be a key publication on the "sociology
   of the Now."

(III:2) 380

Charbonneau, L. 1965. Psychedelic-40.
    Bantam Books, New York.

   Psychedelics in science fiction.
   Psychedelic-40 is PSI-40, the drug
   that gave the "Syndicate" power over
   the minds of people. Thus the Specials,
   who are souped-up syndicate members, set
   up a psychedelic society complete with
   psychedelic nudist colonies, fornication
   bars, and mystical temples of the "Society
   of the Immortal Light."

(III:2) 381

Didion, J. Slouching towards Bethlehem.
    Farrar, Straus & Giroux, Inc., New
    York.

   A varied series of movingly written
   chapters on the quality and nature
   of American life in the late 1960s.
   The title chapter studies the Haight-
   Ashbury scene during summer 1967, the
   first season of flower-children. By
   one of the country's finest journalists.

(III:2) 382

Felton, D., and D. Dalton. 1970. Year of
   the fork, night of the hunter.
   Rolling Stone Magazine, 25 June:24-48.

   An account of the life of Charles Manson,
   culminating in the Sharon Tate tragedy
   of August, 1969. Interesting for its
   explication of Manson's character as a
   product of the counter-culture, showing
   how the ethic of love can be perverted.

(III:2) 383

Fort, J. 1969. The pleasure seekers.
   Grove Press, New York.

   The drug crisis, youth, and society, discussed (according to reviews) in a timely
   and comprehensive manner. Fort is convinced
   that psychoactive drugs, contrary to unenlightened popular belief, provide society
   with a net gain. In extolling their virtues,
   he often flippantly dismisses their dangers
   to the point that the whole argument loses
   force and credibility. A psychiatrist's
   attempt to be "with it" in a book where
   the attempt almost fails.

(III:2) 384

Gardner, H. 1970. Your global alternative:
   communes, experiments, jails, and
   hidey-holes. Esquire September:106-112.

   A listing of and discussion about various
   communal living groups throughout the
   United States. Communes are believed
   by some commentators to be the core unit
   of the drug culture and a prime testing
   ground of its tenets.

(III:2) 385

Gioscia, V. 1969. LSD subcultures: acidoxy versus orthodoxy. Amer. J. Orthopsych. 39:428-436.

The distinguishing characteristics of the LSD subculture are outlined on the basis of data gathered in San Francisco, New York, and London. Some are: "subcultural differentiations", "status", "relevance of experience", "sex", and "religion." The author places these factors within the context of a new alienation model.

(III:2) 386

Gordon, N. 1963. The hallucinogenic drug cult. Reporter. 15 August:35-43.

An attemot to define in layman's terms the assumotions and implications of an emerging counter-culture. The article reflects that particular frenzied journalistic style which was invoked largely to describe the ferment of Timothy Leary's days at Harvard.

(III:2) 387

Greiner, T. 1962. The ethics of drug research on human subjects. J. New Drugs 2:7-22.

Greiner raises questions regarding the misdirection of scientific zeal in the area of human experimentation. His article shrewdly foreshadowed many of the dangerous political consequences of this kind of research, which have been realized only in the last few years.

(III:2) 388

Hall, E. T. 1966. The hidden dimension. Doubleday, New York.

Dr. Hall discusses the territorial imperative of personal space in terms of the "psychic" boundaries of social behavior. His book helps define the nature of social groupings, particularly within the counter-culture.

(III:2)  389

Heinlein, R. A. 1961. Stranger in a strange
 land. Berkley Medallion Books, New York.

 A science fiction novel about a man from
 Mars who functions at a higher level of
 consciousness than normal human beings.
 His reaction to the hypocrisy and ab-
 surdity of many human actions and institutions can be interpreted as an
 allegorical reference to the "hippie"
 viewpoint.

(III:2)  390

Heyman, F. 1972. Methadone maintenance as
 law and order. Society 9:15-75.

 The word "methadone" has become the rallying
 cry for liberal proponents of the argument
 that narcotic addiction should be treated
 as a disease and not as a crime. But in
 this provocative article, the author asserts
 that the word also carries a dangerous,
 right-wing connotation. "The substitution
 of methadone for heroin," she writes, "won't
 rehabilitate the drug addict, but it may
 be used as a method of tranquilizing a
 potentially troublesome ghetto and poor
 white population."

(III:2)  391

Hoffman, A. 1969. Woodstock nation.
 Vintage Books, New York.

 A talk-rock album on paper, purporting
 to be the definitive history of the counter-culture. Hoffman attempts to capture
 and convey the spirit of the movement and
 the ethos of its prime movers. He is
 reasonably successful, providing the
 reader is willing to put up with trun-
 cated sentences and much hand-waving
 about radical politics.

(III:2) 392

Horman, R. E., and A. M. Fox. 1970. Drug awareness. Avon Books, New York.

An anthology, many of the selections in which lack the necessary flair, insight, and factual force to merit a subtitle like "Key Documents on LSD, Marihuana, and the Drug Culture." Of redeeming value are the essays by Joel Fort ("The Semantics and Logic of the Drug Scene"), Kenneth Keniston ("Drug Use and Student Values") and the editors' ("Drug Education Activists, An Innovation"). There is no index.

(III:2) 393

Huxley, A. 1962. Island. Harper and Row, New York.

A utopian novel about a civilization centered around drug-taking. The model for Timothy Leary's psychedelic training center in Zihuatanejo, Mexico is said to have been provided by Island.

(III:2) 394

Keniston, K. 1971. Youth and dissent. Harcourt, Brace Joranovish, New York.

A good, lengthy summary of Keniston's theories on the rise of a dissenting, often radical youthful subculture between 1960 and 1970.

(III:2) 395

Keniston, K. 1971. Young Radicals Harcourt, Brace and World, New York

A Sociological study of radical politics in current generation. This book amphlifies on themes not fully covered in The Uncommitted.

(III:2) 396

Keniston, K. 1965. The uncommitted.
　　Harcourt, Brace and World, Inc., New York.

　　In a stimulating sociological investigation of the causes of alienation from American society, Keniston lucidly analyzes the origins of youthful dissent. Although highly recommended by reviewers, one cannot help but feel that The Uncommitted is ten years out of date. The alienation of youth as it appears to exist in the 70's has already begun to evolve from individualistic alienation and lack of commitment to society toward active, even violent commitment within the emerging sociological species-- the counter-society.

(III:2) 397

Krantz, S. 1968. Deterrents to drug abuse: the role of the law. J. Amer. Med. Assoc. 206:1276-1279.

　　A summary of the historical development of federal and state drug abuse laws in the U.S. The author calls for law enforcement resources to be strengthened following the sensible revision of existing laws.

(III:2) 398

Laing, R. D. 1967. The politics of experience.
　　Ballantine Books, New York.

　　"The life I am trying to grasp is the me who is trying to grasp it." This is part of Laing's message. The other part calls for a realization that people impinge (politically?) upon the individual while he is attempting to grasp life. In between these themes, Laing asserts the kinship between mental illness and the creative expressions of psychedelic culture, of which he and Leary may be competing chief spokesmen.

(III:2) 399

Lasagna, L. 1969. The pharmaceutical revolution and its impact on society. Science 166:1227-1233.

    The author traces the historical development and social impact of what he calls "biopharmaceutical technology" from several centuries B.C. to the present. He sees in this development a continuing struggle between profiteers and public officials for the final say in establishing standards of drug quality.

(III:2) 400

Leary, T. 1968. The politics of ecstasy. Putnam's Sons, New York.

    A "sour grapes" disquisition on why the Establishment cannot and will not accept the new politics of counter-culture.

(III:2) 401

Leary, T., and R. Alpert. 1963. The politics of consciousness expansion. Harvard Rev. 1:33-37.

    Leary and Alpert plead their case, which they feel is being harshly tried by the proponents of strict academe. Several of the themes in this short essay subsequently ballooned in Leary's <u>Politics</u> <u>of</u> <u>Ecstasy</u>.

(III:2) 402

Lennard, H., L. J. Epstein, H. Stein, and D. C. Ranson. 1971. Mystification and drug misuse. Josey-Bars Inc., San Francisco.

    A series of essays addressed to the general proposition that the principal hazard in the use of psychoactive drugs is to surround that use with impenetrable conceptual barriers.

(III:2) 403

Lennard, H. L., L J. Epstein, and M. S. Rosenthal. 1972. The methadone illusion. Science 176:881-884.

An examination of both the cases for and against methadone maintenance. This particular discussion takes the point of view that the "heroin epidemic" is part of an ever increasing "internal pollution" of society through the ubiquitous use of psychoactive drugs. So, the authors contend, any discussion of the methadone question, in order to be meaningful, must address itself to issues beyond the heroin addict.

(III:2) 404

Lindesmith, A. R. 1965. The addict and the law. Indiana University Press, Bloomington, Indiana.

Dr. Lindesmith clarifies the issues involved against a thorough background of internationally-compiled statistics. His prose is forceful and free of self-righteous rhetoric, lending impressive credence to the imperative "Thou shalt not punish disease."

(III:2) 405

Louria, D. B. 1966. Nightmare drugs. Pocket Books, New York.

An example of the alarmist approach to the drug question, even though the author usually qualifies his points. Not helpful for understanding the drug cult and its sociological as well as its biological complexities.

(III:2) 406

Louria, D. B. 1968. The drug scene. McGraw-Hill, New York.

Though Louria is considered an authority, the book is generally unenlightened, superficial and misleading. No index, and only a scanty bibliography.

(III:2) 407

Milbauer, B., and G. Leinwald, eds. 1970. Drugs. Washington Square Press, New York.

A "scare tactics" primer containing abridged articles already published elsewhere, offensive photographs, and irrelevant questions "for further inquiry" at the end of each chapter. Not, as the subtitles suggest, "a searching look at the turned-on world."

(III:2) 408

Mintz, M. 1965. The therapeutic nightmare. Houghton-Mifflin, Boston.

A definitive study "on the roles of the United States Food and Drug Administration, pharmaceutical manufacturers and others in connection with the irrational and massive use of prescription drugs that may be worthless, injurious, or even lethal." Does not treat the uses and misuses of psychedelics.

(III:2) 409

Masters, P., ed. 1970. Playboy panel: the drug revolution. Playboy 17(2):53-74, 200-201.

A round table discussion between Harry Anslinger, William Burroughs, James Coburn, Baba Ram Dass (nee Richard Alpert), Leslie Fiedler, John Finlator, Joseph Oteri, and Alan Watts. On a wide range of topics, fast-moving and flashy. This is an article with an overriding theme that calls for the drug culture to become a political force in contemporary society.

(III:2) 410

National Library of Medicine Literature Searches. 1970. Drug abuse and crime. Dept. of Health, Education and Welfare, U.S. Government Printing Office, Washington, D.C.

A bibliography (L.S. No. 70-75) covering 73 references from January 1967 to December 1969.

(III:2) 411

National Library of Medicine Literature
    Searches. 1970. Mortality of self-
    destructive behavior in drug abuse.
    Dept. of Health, Education and Welfare,
    U.S. Government Printing Office, Wash-
    ington, D.C.

   A bibliography (L.S. No. 70-73) covering
   59 references from January 1967 to
   December 1969.

(III:2) 412

Newitt, J., M. Singer, and H. Kahn. 1971.
    Some speculations on U.S. drug use.
    J. Soc Issues 27:107-122.

   This paper from the Hudson Institute
   addresses itself to the ethical questions that will be raised twenty or
   thirty years from now when drugs will
   be used more for the control of human
   behavior than for "mind expansion."

(III:2) 413

Proger, S., ed. 1968. The medicated society.
    MacMillan, New York.

   The essays offered in this anthology
   document and support the notion that
   the United States--and in a more general
   sense all of western society--has been
   a drug culture long before the advent
   of Leary and Haight-Ashbury.

(III:2) 414

Psychedelic Review, eds. 1964. Editorial.
    Psychedel. Rev. 1:372-377.

   At the end of the editorial is a list
   of 19 articles from popular periodicals
   on the drug scene for the years 1963-64,
   ranging from sober assessments to super-
   cilious expressions of cynicism (according
   to the editors).

(III:2) 415

Roszak, T. 1969. The making of a counter culture. Doubleday, Garden City, New York.

While stressing the need for the survival of the counter culture, Roszak emphasizes the dangers it faces, such as subversion by commercial or political influences. His explanation of the roots of the counter culture (an essentially apolitical dissatisfaction with the problems inherent in technocracy) is excellent, but his attempts at categorizing the mainstreams of counter-cultural thought are considerably less successful.

(III:2) 416

Sheehy, G. 1971. Speed is of the essence. Simon and Schuster, New York.

Somewhat journalistic account of various facets of life among the alienated (e.g. speed-freaks and women alone). The section on speed is basically a long case study in which the author discusses her involvement as friend and conselor to a group of speed freaks.

(III:2) 417

Simmons, J. L., and B. Winograd. 1967. It's a happening. Marc-Laird Publications, Santa Barbara, California.

An early account of the California scene by two young sociologists, written in a sympathetic and disarming style.

(III:2) 418

Slater, P. 1971. The pursuit of loneliness. Beacon Press, Boston.

Discusses loneliness in American life, and the search for community and dependent relationships in a society which stresses fragmentation and independence.

(III:2) 419

Stafford, P. 1971. Psychedelic baby reaches puberty. Praeger Publishers, New York.

An insider views and interviews twenty key figures in the "drug culture", including Allen Ginsberg, Bill Graham, Alan Watts, and Humphrey Osmond. Their testimonies lead the author to conclude what he apparently set out to conclude, namely that psychedelic drugs may have a humanizing and unifying effect on an increasingly technological society which threatens to make the collective nightmare of <u>1984</u>, <u>Animal Farm</u> and <u>Brave New World</u> a reality.

(III:2) 420

Talalay, P., ed. 1964. Drugs in our society. The Johns Hopkins Press, Baltimore.

A comprehensive collection of sociologically-oriented articles in a well-organized anthology. The contributions are factual as well as interpretative and provide numerous bibliographic aids for further study. Topics include: "Drug Costs and the Consumer," "Drug Experiments and the Public Conscience," "The Functions of the Pharmaceutical Industry in Our Society," "The Responsibilities and Problems of Government," and "Social History of American Drug Legislation."

(III:2) 421

Tannebaum, A. J. 1969. Alienated youth. J. Soc. Issues 25:1-146.

A series of papers updating Keniston's study (Ref. #396). Two articles in this symposium are particularly illuminating: Edgar Friedenberg's "Current Patterns of a Generational Conflict" reviews the counterculture scene. He has several paragraphs on contemporary folk-rock. Sanford Reichart offers an additional overview in "A Greater Space in which to Breathe: What Art and Drama Tell Us about Alienation."

(III:2) 422

Walsh, J. 1971. Drug abuse control: policy turns toward rehabilitation. Science 173:32-34.

A news review and commentary on the politics and finances of developing rehabilitation programs, particularly for G.I. addicts.

(III:2) 423

Watts, A. W. 1961. Psychotherapy east and west. Pantheon Books, New York.

Eternity, according to the author, is now, and therefore his book is devoted to exploring how eternity (or, in other words, liberation) is achieved within Eastern and Western culture. Throughout the exploration, Mr. Watts advocates transcendental experience as the ideal escape from repression of the body and from the dull routines of getting and spending that society has imposed upon mankind. The book has been described as a fundamental document in the shaping of the commune culture.

(III:2) 424

Wood, R. W. 1970. Major federal and state narcotics programs and legislation. Crime and Delin. 16:36-56.

A description and evaluation of programs, citing seventy references, including court cases and government documents.

(III:2) 425

Young, J. H. 1961. The toadstool millionaires: A social history of patent medicines in America before federal regulation. Princeton University Press, Princeton.

The development of patent medicines is related to broader trends in health, education, and medical quackery. Dr. Young also offers an enlightening sociological commentary on such subjects as the widespread use and abuse of opiated tonics, syrups and cures two or more generations ago.

(III:2) 426

Zinberg, N. E., and J. A. Robertson. 1972. Drugs and the public. Simon and Schuster, New York.

This book is dedicated almost exclusively to the legal problems presented by current public attitudes to drug use. The reader should note in particular the chapters on drug laws, the cost of drug laws, alternatives to drug control (such as licensing of users), and the "British Experience."

# CHAPTER IV

# Cultural and Philosophic Overviews:

# The Drug Experience

(IV) 427

Abrams, M. H. 1970. The milk of paradise.
    Harper and Row, New York.

A short book of annotated essays intended to explain how DeQuincy, Crabbe, Thompson and Coleridge--four eminent English authors--incorporated the imagery from drug induced dream worlds into their literary creations. Although it was first published in 1934 as Mr. Abram's senior honors thesis, <u>Milk of Paradise</u> is still regarded as one of the few comprehensive studies of the effects of opium in literature, which have appeared since then.

(IV) 428

Adams, J. K. 1963. Psychosis: "experimental" and "real". Psychedel. Rev. 2:121-144.

Psychosis theorized as a sudden and drastic change in cognitive structure. Psychedelics fall into the general scheme as catalysts for the sudden change. Adams supports his arguments with references to classics of Western literature and philosophy. Extensive notes and a detailed bibliography.

(IV) 429

Adams, R. L., and R. J. Fox. 1972.
    Mainlining Jesus: the new trip.
    Society 9:50-56.

This timely essay compares the drug and the Jesus cultures, and the authors conclude that instead of progressing toward adult ethics, the Jesus people, like their counterparts in the drug culture, clutch "tenaciously to childhood morality, with its simplistic black-and-white, right-and-wrong judgements."

(IV) 430

Alexander, M. 1967. The sexual paradise of
    LSD. Brandon House, North Hollywood.

A fanciful look at the sexual power of LSD both as a physiological and a psychic aphrodisiac.

(IV) 431

Barber, T. X. 1970. LSD, marihuana, yoga and hypnosis. Aldine Publishing Company, Chicago.

In this often mentioned critique of the experimental literature, the author traces the relationship between altered states of consciousness produced by drugs and those produced by hypnosis. Although the subject has been discussed in numerous other publications, it is covered most extensively in this paperback monograph, which also includes an extensive bibliography.

(IV) 432

Barron, F. 1958. The psychology of imagination. Sci. Am. 199(3):150-166.

A study of the characteristics of creative individuals working with or without the help of psychoactive drugs.

(IV) 433

Baudelaire, C. 1971. Artificial paradise. Herder and Herder, New York.

This is a new paperback edition of parts of Charles Baudelaire's Les Paradis Artificiels originally published in 1860. Throughout the Artificial Paradise the poet tells how he has penetrated the unknown and attained the infinite with wine and hashish. The book ends with a stirring plea by the poet for achieving without the use of drugs the extraordinary state of consciousness which he had experienced under hashish.

(IV) 434

Bays, G. 1969. The orphic vision. Seer poets from Novalis to Rimbaud. University of Nebraska Press, Lincoln.

The vision of the mystic; the ecstasy of the poet; the delirium of the opium smoker: all are facets of the same intricate diamond, the mind. Prof. Bays documents this hypothesis with detailed analyses of the writings of famous madmen or philosophers-- Plotinus, Swedenborg, Kant--and of seer poets, who all felt the illumination of hashish--Hoffman, Gautier, Baudelaire, Verlaine, Nerval, and Rimbaud.

(IV) 435

Bishop, M. G. 1963. Discovery of love.
Dodd, Mead and Company, New York.

"Bishop's account is notable for clarity, cogency and straightforwardness," writes Humphrey Osmond in the foreword, and so it is. The author shares his doubts and fears about LSD as well as the pleasure he derived from it in his pursuit of "oneness" and love. At the very least, this short novel conveys the impression that psychedelics--like any other social or psychological tools--can be either a boon or a curse, depending on how they are used.

(IV) 436

Bloch, I. 1933. Anthropological studies in the strange sexual practices of all races in all ages, ancient and modern.
Anthropological Press, New York.

An old classic, brimming with tidbits about drugs and sex. The erotic effects of opium are described in special detail.

(IV) 437

Blood, B. P. 1874. The anaesthetic revelation and the gist of philosophy. Amsterdam Press, New York.

An attempt to relate the highest of human thought processes--creative intuition--to the psychic state produced immediately after anesthesia. For Blood, the "anaesthetic revelation" was "a certain survived condition...in which the genius of being is revealed but because it cannot be remembered in the normal condition it is lost altogether...and buried amid the hum of returning common sense, under that epitaph of all illumination: 'this is a dull world!'"

(IV) 438

Boisen, A. 1952. The exploration of the inner world. Harper, New York.

As Robert Mogar points out in Psychedelics, long before the advent of mind drugs, Anton Boisen had reached the conclusion that acute mental illness and sudden revelations, insights, or transformations of character "arise out of a common situation--that of inner conflict and disharmony, accompanied by a keen awareness of ultimate loyalties and unattained possibilities...Where it is unsuccessful or indeterminate it is spoken of as 'insanity.' In those constructive transformations...the individual...is brought into harmony with that which is supreme in his hierarchy of loyalties."

(IV) 439

Braden, W. 1967. The private sea: LSD and the search for God. Quadrangle Books, Chicago.

In this controversial monograph, Braden asserts that the psychedelic experience is predicated upon religious feeling which cannot be part of any organized religion, documenting his case with numerous examples such as that of Christianity, whose traditional values, he claims, are being shaken by forces within psychedelic culture.

(IV) 440

Burroughs, W. 1953. Junkie. Ace Books Inc., New York.

Considered to be a classic. A pitilessly factual and hard-boiled account of the addicts' underworld and its denizens-- the moochers, the fags, the stool pigeons, and the thieves. DeQuincy viewed the wasteland of the addict as dream-fantasy; Burroughs views it as phantasmagoria.

(IV) 441

Burton, R. 1621. The anatomy of melancholy.
    1964 edition, H. Jackson, ed. E. P.
    Dutton & Company, New York.

    A seventeenth century classic in three
    volumes about a state of mind now known
    as manic depression. In volume two,
    Burton cites chemical cures--which date
    back to classical time--for melancholy
    and describes the effects when they "ele-
    vate the mind from the depths of despair."
    Poppy, henbane, mandrake, nightshade,
    and nutmeg are frequently recommended
    for this purpose.

(IV) 442

Castaneda, C. 1969. The teachings of Don
    Juan: A Yanqui way of knowledge.
    Ballantine Books, New York.

    A startling first person account of the
    author's plunge into a Central American
    drug cult based on the use of peyote,
    Datura, and sacred mushrooms. The detailed
    descriptions of hallucinogenic experiences
    and ceremonial rites give the book exceptional
    interest from both cultural and psychological
    perspectives.

(IV) 443

Castaneda, C. 1971. A separate reality:
    further conversations with Don Juan.
    Simon and Schuster, New York.

    A sequel to The Teachings of Don Juan
    and dedicated to the same theme.

(IV) 444

Clark, W. H. 1969. Chemical ecstasy: psychedelic drugs and religion. Sheed and Ward, New York.

Dr. Clark, professor emeritus of the psychology of religion at the Andover Newton Theological Seminary, devoted this book to the drawing of parallels "advisedly, deliberately, and thoughtfully" toward the discussion of ecstasy in religion. "As a scholar," he summarizes in the concluding chapter, "I have learned at least as much, though not more, from my six 'trips' as I have from all the plodding study in my field of the psychology of religion." For

those not interested in religion, Dr. Clark's book will serve as a succinct historical survey of drug-induced and non-drug-induced experiences, and as the best available account of Timothy Leary's rise and fall at Harvard.

(IV) 445

Davy, H. 1800. Researches chemical and philosophical, chiefly concerning nitrous oxide of deohlogisticated nitrous air and its respiration. Bristol and Cottle, St. Paul's Churchyard.

Davy ranks among the first to have undertaken active experimentation with psychoactive materials. His observations on the effects of nitrous oxide are reputed to have influenced other 19th century luminaries interested in the same subject, including De Quincey (1822), Moreau (1845), Benjamin Paul Blood (1874) and William James (1902). The significance of Davy's book is perhaps best exemplified by a few sentences the young scientist wrote on

December 26, 1799, after a self-experiment with nitrous oxide: "I felt a sense of tangible extension highly pleasurable in every limb. My visual impressions were dazzling and apparently magnified...I lost all connection with external things; trains of vivid visible images rapidly passed through my mind and even connected with words in such a manner as to produce perceptions perfectly novel...nothing exists but thoughts! --the universe is composed of impressions, ideas, pleasures, and pains."

(IV) 446

De Felice, P. 1936. Poisons sacres, iuresse divine. Editions Albin, Paris.

A cautious investigation of the relationship between religious experience and various hallucinogenic substances throughout history. The text, in French, is considered to be a classic.

(IV) 447

De Quincey, T. 1822. Confessions of an English opium-eater. Oxford University Press, London.

One of the more often cited "modern" accounts of the euphoric state produced by opiates. De Quincey, a noted author of the Romantic period, had been taking laudanum (opiated alcohol) since 1804. He was an admirer of Wordsworth and Coleridge, who also was a chronic user of the drug. Other works reflecting De Quincey's experiences are Susoiria de Profundis and The English Mail Coach.

(IV) 448

De Ropp, R. S. 1968. The master game. Dell Publishing Company, New York.

De Ropp analyzes the levels of consciousness through which human beings act out their lives on the stage of life. Some attain the necessary wisdom and insight to do so effectively by means of drugs. Others must resort to mysticism, and still others to madness. The "master game" can be played in many ways, but in the author's opinion, the best ways are those built upon psychic experiences readily identifiable as non-drug analogues to the psychedelic experience.

(IV) 449

Durr, R. A. 1970. Poetic vision and the psychedelic experience. Syracuse University Press, Syracuse, New York.

Dr. Durr examines the similarities between the psychic states induced by psychedelic drugs and the visionary experiences related by the imaginative poets--Blake, Coleridge, Wordsworth, Vaughn, and Traherne.

(IV) 450

Ebin, D. 1965. The drug experience. Grove Press, New York.

A series of essays presenting first-person accounts of addicts, writers, scientists, historians and noted creative personalities. Bibliographic notes. This is a rare book.

(IV) 451

Eliade, M. 1964. Shamanism: archaic techniques of ecstasy. Pantheon, New York.

Professor Eliade documents this religion of northern Asia and Europe characterized by the ardent belief in a noumenal world of gods, demons and ancestral spirits. In the pursuit of mystical ecstasy under Shamanism, the Ural-Altaic peoples are reputed to have often resorted to intoxication through hemp, mushrooms, or narcotics.

(IV) 452

Erikson, M. H. 1965. A special inquiry with
    Aldous Huxley into the nature and character
    of various states of consciousness.
    Amer. J. Clin. Hypnosis. 8:14-33.

   This interview with Aldous Huxley by a
   noted hypnotist stresses parallels between
   the psychedelic state and its non-drug
   analogues, hypnosis in particular. Huxley's
   view of himself as a visionary--with or
   without drugs--dominates the discussion.

(IV) 453

Farber, L. H. 1968. Ours is the addicted
    society. Rev. Exist. Psychol. Psychiat.
    8:5-15.

   The author underscores the modern
   "disability of will" as the cause of
   moral and intellectual decline in
   Western society. "It was only a
   question of time before man, in his
   desperation, would locate divinity
   in drugs and on that artificial rock
   build his church."

(IV) 454

Farnsworth, D. 1963. Hallucinogenic agents.
    J. Amer. Med. Assoc. 185:878-880.

   An example of a conservative physician's
   viewpoint toward drugs. Dr. Farnsworth
   deplores the making of a psychedelic
   culture on the college campus.

(IV) 455

Finlator, J. 1968. The drug syndrome in the
    affluent society. J Forensic Sci. 13:
    293-301.

   The point of view of the law enforcer is
   advanced in this article. The drug syndrome
   is viewed as a logical consequence of the
   attitudes fostered by a society that can
   buy its way out of everything--from law
   to reality itself.

(IV) 456

Fischer, R. 1968. Space-time co-ordinates of excited and tranquilized states. Pages 33-51 in Psychiatry and art. S. Karger, Basel.

Fischer brings his discussion of drug experiences to bear directly on the relationship between psychiatry and art. The two disciplines complement each other, he notes, because both deal intimately with cerebral, sensory, and physical space.

(IV) 457

Fischer, R. 1971. A cartography of the ecstatic and meditative states. Science 174:897-904.

An expanded version of Professor Fischer's previous article in Science on the perception-hallucination continuum with particular reference to a new dimension: the perception-meditation continuum. The role of hard and soft drugs within this latter framework is discussed in detail.

(IV) 458

Fuller, J. G. 1968. The day of St. Anthony's fire. MacMillan, New York.

An account of the tragedy that occurred in 1951 in the French town of Pont-Saint-Espirit, where the entire population apparently ingested LSD accidentally as a result of fermented rye ergot in the bread supply.

(IV) 459

Furst, P. T. 1972. Flesh of the gods. Praeger, New York.

Ten essays on the ritual use of hallucinogens, primarily in Western primitive cultures. The book includes contributions by well-known authors, such as Schultes, Wasson, and La Barre--who have written extensively on the role of drugs in relgion and ecstasy. The book emerged from a public lecture series at the University of California at Los Angeles in the spring of 1970.

(IV) 460

Ginsberg, A., and W. Burroughs. 1963.
    The yage letters. City Lights Books,
    San Francisco.

    Burroughs set out in 1953 to find yage
    (ayahuasca or caapi), a hallucinogenic
    plant found in South American jungles.
    He wrote to Ginsberg of his overdose
    nightmares, and Ginsberg replied seven
    years later after trying yage in Peru.
    The correspondence is about their mutual
    desire to discover a chemical exit from
    the mind.

(IV) 461

Gotz, I. L. 1970. The psychedelic teacher.
    Westminster Press, Philadelphia.

    An explanation of the drug culture
    phenomenon as a consequence of the
    failure of the American educational
    system at providing a viable alter-
    native to the mystical ecstasy young
    people think they can attain through
    drugs. That alternative should be the
    psychedelic teacher--a mystic in the
    classroom.

(IV) 462

Gustaitis, R. 1969. Turning on.
    Signet Books, New York.

    Ostensibly a report on America's new
    psychic frontiers, appreciated by a
    liberated woman (the author), the book
    covers a multitude of current fads, but
    contains little of substance or signifi-
    cance compared to others of its genre.
    Ms. Gustaitis wishes the reader to believe
    she is the counterpart of Timothy Leary.

(IV) 463

Hayter, A. 1969. Opium and the romantic
    imagination. University of California
    Press, Berkeley.

    Literary criticism on references to
    opiates and sleeping potions in stories
    ranging from the Arabian Nights to The
    Moonstone. The authors discussed in
    greatest detail are Poe, Coleridge, Crabbe,
    Keats, and Thomas de Quincey.

(IV) 464

Headlee, R. 1967. Fantasy and disease.
   Exist. Psychiat. 1:440-457.

   A "theoretical attempt to make more
   constructive use of the existing knowledge of the fantasy process in the
   study of the nature of disease." The
   author's findings may be compared to
   similar ones obtained from analyses of
   the "drug experience."

(IV) 465

Hennell, T. 1938. The witnesses.
   Davies, London.

   A gripping account of the author's
   schizophrenic experience. Commentators
   on the psychedelic scene have often
   likened Hennell's tortured chronicle
   to a protracted LSD trip.

(IV) 466

Herz, S. 1968. Behavioral patterns in sex
   and drug use on three campuses: implications for education and society.
   Psychiat. Quart. 42:258-271.

   As with so many other complex sociological
   phenomena, no fast holding causative relationships can be identified, and this
   assertion is particularly true with regard
   to the subject of drug use and sex. Upon
   considerable deliberation, the authors
   conclude that the Kama Sutra oil orgy
   and the pot party in some instances are
   related causally and in others, not at
   all. At best, no generalizations can be
   made.

(IV) 467

Hesse, H. 1949. The bead game.
   Holt, Rhinehart and Winston, New York.

   Hesse explained in 1955 why he wrote the book: "In opposition to the present world I had to show the realm of mind and of spirit, show it as real and unconquerable; thus my work became a Utopia. The image was projected into the future, and to my surprise the world of Castalia emerged almost by itself." Castalia, "the future society of mystic game players"--"the players with pearls of glass"--received enthusiastic endorsement in a book review by Leary and Metzner.

   ("Herman Hesse: Poet of the Interior Journey." Psychedelic Review 2:167-182. 1963) These two psychedelic seers helped set up the Castalia Foundation, Millbrook, New York to promote the expansion of awareness.

(IV) 468

Hesse, H. 1922. Siddhartha. 1951 ed.
   New Directions, New York.

   Timothy Leary and Ralph Metzner wrote once about Hesse's novel that those who have taken one of the psychedelic drugs may recognize Siddhartha's visions as classic LSD sequences. Siddhartha, the protagonist of the novel, sought to attain cosmic one-upmanship--more enlightenment than Buddha himself. (Similar themes under a different setting are also expressed in Steppenwolf by the same author.)

(IV) 469

Hollander, L. 1970. If they're into rock, study rock. New York Times. August 9, Section II, p. 11.

   The author analytically relates music appreciation in the young to some of the major cultural questions facing the whole of society.

(IV) 470

Hughes, H. M., ed. 1961. The fantastic lodge. Houghton-Mifflin, Boston.

Subtitled "the autobiography of a girl drug addict", this account transcribed from original recordings can be read in a variety of ways: as a psychiatric case study, as an account of the use of narcotics, or as a sociological document based upon an individual point of view.

(IV) 471

Huxley, A. 1964. The doors of perception and Heaven and hell. Harper and Row, New York.

Two classic works comprising observations, musings and speculations by the author concerning the psychedelic experience and the future of Western culture. Huxley suggests that the reality of the mind can be grasped only with the aid of psychedelic drugs, which bring knowledge, wisdom, and a vision of God, or at least of his Paradise. The Doors of Perception is fast becoming the most-quoted single work on the subject.

(IV) 472

Huxley, J. 1962. Psychometabolism. J. Nueropsychiat. 3(1):S1-S14.

Sir Julian's classic essay reflects the ambivalences of the biologist who attempts to answer existential questions about the mind. The essay examines how the developing human being can integrate his interior life by turning towards any one of many "psychometabolic" activities, such as the arts, mysticism, or psychedelia.

(IV) 473

James, W. 1911. A pluralistic mystic.
    Pages 369-411 in W. James, Memories
    and studies. Longmans, New York.

    "Not for the ignoble vulgar do I write
    this article, but only for those dialectic-
    mystic souls who have an irresistable
    taste, acquired or native, for higher
    flights of metaphysics." With these
    words, James lauched his defense of
    Benjamin Paul Blood and argued much in
    the same vein that the secrets of the
    mind can only be grasped when the mundane
    is transcended through natural or chemical
    ecstasy.

(IV) 474

James, W. 1902. The varieties of religious
    experience. Modern Library, New York.

    A comprehensive attempt to bring the
    states of trans-normal consciousness
    into the mainstream of philosophy.
    James includes a discussion of his famous
    experiments with nitrous oxide as a faci-
    litating agent for the production of mysti-
    cal states and experiences. The chapters
    on "Religion and Neurology" and "Mysticism"
    are especially timely.

(IV) 475

Johnson, C. E. 1967. Mystical force of the
    nightshade. Int. J. Neuropsychiat. 3:
    268-275.

    The author presents an abstracted history
    of the use and results of Datura and cites
    his personal experiences with the drug plant.
    Datura otherwise known as Jamestown weed or
    Jimson weed, is one of the most common
    psychoactive plants in the world, ranging
    throughout subtropical Africa, Asia and
    the entire American continent, where it
    has found wide use within religious or
    orgiastic rituals.

(IV) 476

Kaolan, B., ed. 1964. The inner world of
    mental illness. Harper, New York.

This reader is recommended by R. D. Laing,
Bernard Aaronson, and Humphrey Osmond. The
articles presented emphasize the much-
quoted observation from Laing's The Politics
of Experience that madness need not be all
breakdown. "It may also be breakthrough."

(IV) 477

Kris, E. 1952. Psychoanalytic explorations
    in art. 1964 ed. Schocken Books, New York.

The origin of the normal creative urge in
man is examined, in addition to the questions
of psychotic and schizophrenic art. A detailed
bibliography is included and bears numerous
references to pertinent Freudian and non-
Freudian psychoanalytic studies.

(IV) 478

La Barre, W. 1970. Old and New World narcotics:
    a statistical question and an ethnological
    reply. Econ. Bot. 24:73-80.

This short essay presents a succinct summarizing discussion of Pan-American Paleo-
Indian basic culture. In it, Professor La
Barre supports Schultes' thesis that the
American Indians were culturally motivated
to seek out psychoactive plant substances.
"American Indians," he writes, "sought the
mystic visionary experience; their epistemo-
logical touchstone for reality was direct
psychic experience of the forces in nature,
not a sophisticated critique that seeks to
rid experience of subjective elements; and

they...sought, under this religio-cultural
inspiration the actively psychedelic
drugs to ensure this state." The author
cites his previous publications and those
of Dr. Schultes' as supportive evidence.

(IV) 479

Laing, R. D. 1965. Transcendental experience in relation to religion and psychosis. Psychedel. Rev. 6:7-15.

Laing finds a one-to-one correspondence: "Madness need not be all breakdown. It is also breakthrough." Similar thoughts are to be found in his 1967 book, The Politics of Experience.

(IV) 480

Latendresse, J. 1968. Masturbation and its relation to addiction. Rev. Exist. Psychol. Psychiat. 8:16-27.

A cultural and literary examination of the pleasure principle and its relationship to self-abuse. Latendresse's analogy between drug addiction and masturbation is a particularly ingenious one, but has not attracted much attention in the area of public concern over the drug culture.

(IV) 481

Leary, T. 1968. High priest. World Publishing Company, New York.

The psychedelic bible according to Leary, archetypal Lotus-eater, begins "In the beginning was the TURN ON, the flash, the illumination, the electric trip, the sudden bolt of energy that starts the new system. The TURN ON was God." Highly recommended if only because it represents the collective consciousness and collaborative work of such notables as Gordon Wasson, Aldous Huxley, Allen Ginsberg, Ralph Metzner, and Richard Alpert (now Baba Ram Das) who all influenced Leary's trip-by-trip progression through life from January 1959 to June 1962.

(IV) 482

Leary, T., R. Metzner, and R. Alpert. 1964. The psychedelic experience. University Books, New Hyde Park, New York.

A handbook for the proper use of psychedelic drugs according to the sacred rituals and traditions preserved in the Tibetan Book of the Dead. The authors attempt to provide a framework for the integration of psychedelic culture into the sphere of eastern mysticism.

(IV) 483

Leary, T. 1966. Psychedelic prayers. Poet's Press, Kerhonkson, New York.

Prayers, hymns, and incantations heavily influenced by oriental mysticism. To bridge the oceans between the ancient and sacred and the modern and secular, Leary also exalts DNA, the master molecule of heredity. Several selections are undeniably powerful.

(IV) 484

Leary, T. 1964. The religious experience: its production and interpretation. Psychedel. Rev. 1:325-346.

Leary writes as a theologian, addressing himself to the question of ultimate power, life, human destiny and the ego. He concludes that from 40 to 90 per cent of psychedelic subjects report intense religious experiences.

(IV) 485

Lewis, B. 1970. The sexual power of marihuana. Ace Books, New York.

The myth that marihuana may be an aphrodisiac has floated around for decades without receiving systematic attention. Addressing herself to it, the author explores the question of marihuana in sexuality, frigidity, marriage and infidelity. She concludes that many, if not all, of the alleged sexually stimulatory properties of the drug are elicited by the set and setting in which it is used.

(IV) 486

Lilly, J. C. 1972. Programming and metaprogramming in the human biocomputer. Julian Press, New York.

This expanded second edition of a previous book heralds a new age of jargon in which the collective fields of biophysics, neurophysiology, computer theory, electronics and neuroanatomy are integrated (that is, metaprogrammed) into a whole new approach to the study of consciousness. Dr. Lilly asserts that the human mind is a biocomputer with 13 billion active elements and he describes the intricate process by which its mode of functioning can be understood better through the use of LSD.

(IV) 487

Lystad, M. H. 1972. Social alienation: a review of current literature. Sociol. Quart. 13:90-113.

This paper reviews the alienation literature for the last decade, and presents a distillation of over 200 cited publications under four subject headings: "Theoretical and Methodological Issues," "Alienation and Social Structure," "Alienation and Culture Change," and "Alienation and Psychological Disturbance." There are numerous references to the role of alienation in the drug culture.

(IV) 488

Maclay, W. S., and E. Guttman. 1945. Mescaline hallucinations in artists. Arch. Neurol. Psychiat. 45:30-37.

An invaluable reference for study of the shadowy area between the artist's idea and reality, particularly with regard to the effects of an hallucinogen on his ability to perceive his surroundings.

(IV) 489

Maris, R. W. 1971. Deviance as therapy: the paradox of the self-destructive female. J. Health Soc. Behav. 12:113-124.

The author contends after reviewing the theories of Durkheim, Merton and Erikson that drug abuse, along with suicide attempts and sexual deviance are often therapeutic for the individual as well as being useful for maintaining normative boundaries in the larger, non-deviant community.

(IV) 490

Marsh, R. P. 1965. Meaning and the mind-drugs. ETC 22:408-230.

A controversial article relating the psychedelic experience to the achievement of Platonic ideals. Marsh claims that man under LSD comes up against that part of his inner world "where meanings are made, where the patterning process operates in its pure form."

(IV) 491

Masters, R. E. L. 1962. Forbidden sexual behavior and morality. Julian Press, New York.

The book is cited here because of its fourth chapter titled "Sex and Forbidden Drugs: Mescaline and Other Aphrodisiacs," (90 pages). The author discusses the role of opium, heroin, morphine, cocaine, marihuana and the psychedelics in love-making throughout history and under various cultural settings. Several paragraphs are devoted to drugs and the witches' sabbath.

(IV) 492

Masters, R. E. L., and J. Houston, eds. 1968.
   Psychedelic art. Grove Press, New York.

   A collection of essays of a unique nature,
   assembling information on the entire
   spectrum of psychedelic art ranging from
   simple introspection characterized by
   veiled religious imagery, to the most
   complex, confused expressions designed
   to overstimulate the senses. Numerous
   examples from the arts help clarify even
   the more esoteric arguments presented.

(IV) 493

Masters, R. E. L., and J. Houston. 1966.
   The varieties of psychedelic experience.
   Holt, Rinehart and Winston, New York.

   An interpretative study based on first-
   hand observations of 206 drug sessions
   and upon interviews with an additional
   214 subjects who took LSD in a variety
   of settings. The most controversial
   chapters relate to "Psyche and Symbol"
   and to "Religions and Mystical Experience."
   The book is highly recommended in academic
   circles.

(IV) 494

Maupin, E. W. 1965. Zen Buddhism: a psychological
   review. Psychedel. Rev. 5:59-97.

   Although not intended as such, the article
   appears to the reader as an erudite
   rationalization for psychedelic use by
   Westerners who cannot practice Zen. Includes a complete bilbliography supporting
   the author's assertions.

(IV) 495

McGlothlin, W. H., ed. 1971.
   Chemical comforts of man: the future.
   J. Soc. Issues 27:1-147.

   A collection of articles by eleven
   different authors. It is dedicated to
   the proposition that drug use and the
   associated social policy of the future
   "are likely to be determined by various
   other forces which shape society--political
   philosophy, social stability, psychopharmacological advances, and the requirements
   for individual productivity."

(IV) 496

McWhinne, H. J. 1970. Chemical agents for behavior change: "creative, psychotic, and ecstatic states"--some implications for drug education. Brit. J. Addict. 65:123-127.

The purpose of this significant contribution to the study of "chemical ecstasy" is three-fold: 1) to review the research evidence accumulated over the past three years in support of the claim that hallucinogenic drugs aid in creativity; 2) to critically examine the philosophical and value issues of the current drug culture; and 3) to speculate on the educational implications of and the problems generated by the use of drugs among young people in secondary schools.

(IV) 497

Metzner, R., ed. 1968. The ecstatic adventure. MacMillan, New York.

A collection of essays worth reading for the articles by Flofeld ("Consciousness, Energy, Bliss") and Schacter ("The Conscious Ascent of the Soul"), which demonstrate the influence of psychedelics on the production of religious experiences in the Buddhist and Jewish traditions, respectively.

(IV) 498

Metzner, R., and T. Leary. 1966. On programming psychedelic experience. Psychedel. Rev. 9: 5-19.

Typical Leary esoterica: how to use audio-visual techniques plus LSD to promote Tantra, the Buddhist doctrine which teaches that the development of self-understanding has to start with the physical body.

(IV) 499

Mills, J. 1966. The panic in needle park. Farrar, Straus and Giroux, New York.

"Both fiction and fact", according to the author, about pushers, pimps, whores, and heroin in the inner city. A study of the existential setting of the addict.

(IV) 500

Mogar, R. E. 1965. The psychedelic drugs and human potentialities. Pages 324-348 in Explorations in human potentialities, H. Otto, ed. Charles C. Thomas, Springfield, Illinois.

An extensive review devoted to demonstrating that from a clinical point of view LSD may be seen as a beneficial drug that facilitates accurate perception and insight whereas from a laboratory point of view it may be considered to be a dangerous poison capable of stimulating psychotic behavior. Mogar feels too much attention has been focused on the latter view. The subject of LSD is further discussed in the context of modern psychiatric practice.

(IV) 501

Moreau, J. 1845. Du haschisch et de l'alienation mentale. Etudes psychologigues. Librairie de Fortin, Masson, et Cie, Paris.

Moreau's phamphlet, in the tradition of Davy and de Quincey, stands as a historic contribution to the study of psychoactive drugs as chemical guides to the workings of the "insane" mind. Moreau belonged to Le Club des Haschischins, founded by Theophile Gautier, and there befriended Victor Hugo, Honore de Balzac, Gerard de Nerval, and Charles Baudelaire.

(IV) 502

Ouspensky, P. D. 1922. Tertium organum. A key to the enigmas of the world. Alfred A. Knopf, New York.

Ouspensky, the last of the latter day mystics, fascinated the estranged New York intelligentsia of the twenties with his philosophical ramblings. These are of interest because they culminate in a statement regarding the kinship between mysticism and vision and the mystical states produced by narcotics.

(IV) 503

Penner, W. 1972. Hippies' attraction to mysticism. Adolescence 26:199-210.

The author calls this essay a study on how hippies search for personal fulfillment. In that capacity it is an essay of limited usefulness except for a valuable 27 entry bibliography which thoroughly covers the role of mysticism in the counterculture.

(IV) 504

Plato. 427-347 B.C. The laws. Book I. Translated by R. G. Bury. 1952. Harvard University Press, Cambridge. 646A-650B.

In a dialogue on the subject of good and bad laws Plato comments through his protagonists on the role of mental states, the effects of alcohol and drug-induced psychological immunization. It has been suggested by Paul Friedlander (Plato: An Introduction. 1958. Pantheon Books, New York.) that Plato had first-hand experience with psychedelic potions as an initiate into the Eleusinian mysteries. According to the editors of the Psychedelic Review, this "passage anticipates by 2000 years important modern concepts."

(IV) 505

Prince, R., and C. Savage. 1966. Mystical states and the concept of regression. Psychedel. Rev. 8:59-75.

An article on the phenomenology of the infantile state which is approximated by the withdrawal into a psychotic or psychedelic state. A discussion by Walter Houston Clark follows. The 33-item bibliography is mostly on religion, mysticism, and the preconscious foundations of human experience.

(IV) 506

Psychedelic Review, eds. 1963. The subjective after-effects of psychedelic experiences: a summary of four recent questionnaire studies. Psychedel. Rev. 1:1.

First-hand information on the nature of the creative impulses elicited by a psychedelic drug experience.

(IV) 507

Ray, O. S. 1972. Drugs, society and human behavior. C. V. Mosky Company, St. Louis.

Originally the content of this book was material for a course taught at Vanderbilt University. The 15 chapters provide background and basic knowledge about drugs in addition to historical commentary. The author believes that drug use is very much a part of mankind's cultural history and that some of our principal scientific and technological advances have resulted directly from the push for more and newer psychoactive drugs.

(IV) 508

Rockey, M., and R. Fischer. 1969. An interpretation of the aesthetic experience of non-artists under psilocybin. Proc. 5th Int. Congr. Psychopathol. and Artistic Expression. Excerpta Medica Foundation, Paris.

Rockey and Fischer studied the aesthetic experience of non-artists under the influence of psilocybin and found an intensification of already existing personality traits in general and of aesthetic experience in particular.

(IV) 509

Roseman, B. 1963. LSD: The age of mind. Wilshire Book Company, Hollywood.

Mr. Roseman's semi-autobiographical analysis of psychedelic culture begins with a poem leading a prose discussion of mysticism, religious freedom, hypnosis and legends. His attempt to integrate bits and pieces of intellectual history lapses into a fragmentary account of one man's vision, and produces a quaint book (hand-lettered in italic script).

(IV) 510

Sauri, J. J. 1969. The world of hallucination. Exist. Psychiat. 7:91-97.

An impressionistic overview of the literary man's attempt to deal in historical terms with the phenomenon of hallucination.

(IV) 511

Schwartz, B. N. 1968. Psychedelic art. Arts Magazine. April:39-41.

Schwartz defines psychedelic art as "the surrealism of our technological age." The article appeared prior to the publication of Masters' and Houston's monograph on psychedelic art.

(IV) 512

Smith, H. 1964. Do drugs have religious import?
   J. Phil. 61:517-530.

   Professor Smith defends Aldous Huxley's
   position in The Doors of Perception.
   "The conclusion to which evidence currently points," he writes, "would seem
   to be that chemicals can aid the religious
   life, but only where set within a context
   of faith."

(IV) 513

Stace, W. T., ed. 1960. The teachings of the
   mystics. New American Library, New York.

   Selections from Eastern and Western sources
   emphasize the ecstasy with which mystics
   of all ages and cultures have regarded
   their place in the universe.

(IV) 514

Stafford, P. G., and B. H. Golightly. 1967.
   LSD: the problem-solving psychedelic.
   Award Books, New York.

   LSD as panacea. The authors support their
   arguments with excerots of case histories
   and other data that demonstrate the enhancement of human potentialities by
   psychedelics. This book was acclaimed
   by reviews in Psychedelic Review.

(IV) 515

Taqi, S. 1969. Approbation of drug usage in
   rock and roll music. Bull. Narcotics 21:
   29-35.

   A short history of the rock-drug phenomenon,
   what it comprises, and how it came about.
   The author cites thirty or more songs by
   Bob Dylan, Donovan, the Beatles, Rolling
   Stones, Jefferson Airplane, Eric Burdon,
   Country Joe and the Fish, Jimi Hendrix,
   Steppenwolf and others. The conclusion
   to be drawn from an analysis of the lyrics
   is that music can touch the mind only if
   the music is rock and the mind is altered.

(IV) 516

Taqi, S. 1971. Treatment of drug usage in some examples of modern English writing. Bull. Narcotics 23(2):17-31.

A literary survey of both soft and hard drug abuse as a theme in serious novels, popular fiction, thriller fiction, and drug-oriented poetry since World War II. A bibliography of 34 pertinent novels follows the text of this essay.

(IV) 517

Taylor, R. 1970. Baba Ram Dass shares his experiences. Boston Globe Sunday Magazine. 14 June:16-25.

Short but informative biography of a man who is rapidly emerging as an important influence on the counter-culture. The article provides valuable information about Dr. Alpert's switch from LSD to mysticism in the oriental style.

(IV) 518

Van Kaam, A. 1968. Addiction and existence. Rev. Exist. Psychol. Psychiat. 8:54-64.

This study describes the origin, structure and function of the "addictive" personality, and contrasts it to other personality types. Another comprehensive piece by the author of several well-known monographs, including Religion and Personality and The Art of Existential Counseling.

(IV) 519

Wakefield, D., A. Harrison, and A. Huxley. 1963. The pros and cons, history and future possibilities of vision-inducing psychochemicals. Playboy November:84.

Written with flair and Huxley's usual sense of vision, practically every sentence reflects the enthusiasm which characterized the intellectual supporters of psychedelia in the early sixties.

(IV) 520

Watts, A. W. 1961. Psychotherapy east and west.
    Ballantine Books, New York.

   Mr. Watts' book is often regarded as a
   successful attempt at the difficult task
   of explaining Eastern thought to Western
   man in popular terms. Extremely important
   to an understanding of the counter-culture,
   which turns to the East for direction on
   many philosophical issues.

(IV) 521

Watts, A. 1962. The joyous cosmology.
    Random House, Inc., New York.

   A fanciful and poetical description of
   the psychedelic state. Watts writes of
   the cosmic awareness often experienced
   under the influence of hallucinogens.

(IV) 522

Weil, A. T. 1972. Natural mind.
    Houghton-Mifflin, Boston.

   Dr. Weil advances and documents the
   suggestion that the pharmacological
   action of the hallucinogens may con-
   stitute only a neutral stimulus to
   the brain. It can be interpreted
   positively or negatively depending
   on the social-psychological, idio-
   syncratic or cultural situation of
   the user.

(IV) 523

Weil, G. M., R. Metzner, and T. Leary, 1965.
    The psychedelic reader. University Books,
    New Hyde Park, New York.

   A collection of articles from the early
   issues of Psychedelic Review, including
   contributions by Gordon Wasson, Richard
   Schultes, Sir Julian Huxley, Alan Watts,
   and Timothy Leary and Ralph Metzner's
   book review on "Herman Hesse: Poet of
   the Interior Journey." The selections
   either celebrate the drug culture or
   rationalize its attractiveness to
   modern man.

(IV) 524

Wentz-Evans, W. 1960. The Tibetan Book of the Dead. Oxford University Press, London.

> The best current translation of this volume of unknown origin which, according to Leary, must be interpreted as a guide to the spiritual death encountered in the deep psychedelic experience.

(IV) 525

Westhues, K. 1972. Hippiedom 1970: some tentative hypotheses. Sociol. Quart. 13:81-89.

> An essay in partial defense of the term "hippie" as an accurate description of an identity as stable as that of a Christian monk. The writings of 26 experts on the sociology of hippiedom are reviewed in this essay and used to support the author's assertions that the hippie movement is not antinomian, that it is pleasure-affirming, and that it is counter-cultural rather than political.

(IV) 526

Wolfe, T. 1968. The electric kool-aid acid test. Farrar, Straus and Giroux, New York.

> A flashy, journalistic account of Ken Kesey and the beginnings of the west coast drug movement, attempting to convey the nature of various drug experiences; its greater import is as a document in the history of an emergent sub-culture.

(IV) 527

Zaehner, R. C. 1961. Mysticism, sacred and profane. Oxford University Press, New York.

> A monograph held in high esteem by the editors of Psychedelic Review. It documents the origins and history of mysticism. The author partly contends that hallucinogens may be able to elicit pantheistic or monistic types of religion, but cannot be said to stimulate a theistic religious experience.

(IV) 528

Zilboorg, G. 1935. The medical man and the witch during the Renaissance. John Hopkins Press, Baltimore.

Dr. Zilboorg discusses in Chapter II the life and work of Johann Weyer, whom he calls the founder of modern psychiatry. Weyer's treatise De Praestigiis Demonum criticizes the well known Malleus Maleficarum of 1489, a document summarizing the Inquisition's official findings about witches and sorcerers. Weyer tirelessly points out that the behavior of these outcasts from society need not be attributed to sin or to possession by the devil but to the chronic use on their part of concoctions containing belladonna, opium, henbane, hashish and other psychoactive substances.

(IV) 529

Zilboorg, G. 1941. A history of medical psychology. W. W. Norton and Company, New York.

A general, systematic survey of the topic, but Dr. Zilboorg pays particular attention to men like Weyer and Magnan who addressed their scientific inquiries toward that particular form of consciousness generated by the use of psychoactive drugs.

# APPENDIX I

This appendix is intended to provide a summary of information about drugs. But before proceeding to the descriptions of the drugs themselves certain terms need to be defined:

"Tolerance" — The state in which the body has built up a resistance to a drug so that increasing amounts of the drug have to be taken to achieve the desired effect.

"Physical dependence" — The state in which the constant presence of a drug in the body is necessary for the continued normal functioning of the body. If the drug is withdrawn certain physical reactions, sometimes violent, take place.

"Habituation" (psychological dependence) — The state in which an individual needs a drug psychologically but is not physically dependent on it.

"Addiction" — The state in which tolerance, physical dependence, and habituation have been built up to a particular drug.

# APPENDIX I

Alcohol

Action and mechanism: The drug acts exclusively as a depressant of the central nervous system. Initially it affects consciousness and coordination, then respiration and circulation. Its mode of action at the synapse is not known in detail, although evidence exists to suggest that alcohol may depress nerve impulse transmission in isolated nerve cells. Its fundamental mode of action appears to be an interference with energy production and utilization in a wide variety of tissues and organs.

Uses: Occasionally used medicinally as a tranquilizer. Otherwise used as a drink to provide social comfort.

Dangers: Excessive use causes extensive damage to the nervous system, the liver, and the kidney. Single overdoses (in the vicinity of half a pint) may be fatal.

Potential for psychological dependence: high
Potential for physiological dependence: high
Potential for tolerance: moderate

Preparations: Miscellaneous distillates from fermented grains, grapes, berries, or roots. The effective doses are variable.

APPENDIX I

## Amphetamines

Action and mechanism: Potent cerebral stimulants, causing wakefulness, heightened mood, talkativeness, and random motor activity. Their mode of action is not understood.

Uses: a) Produce wakefulness, reverse fatigue and depressed psychic states; b) as respiratory stimulants in patients suffering from barbiturate poisoning; c) in the treatment of obesity.

Dangers: Overdoses cause nervousness, insomnia, and in extreme cases hallucinations and delirium.

Potential for psychological dependence: high
Potential for physiological dependence: none
Potential for tolerance: high, as much as 2 grams per day may be taken.

Preparations: Benzedrine, Dexedrine, Methedrine, Desoxyn. Most addicts begin with low doses of amphetamines taken orally, (10 to 30 mg) and slowly increase their dosage up to 150 to 250 mg daily.

## Antidepressants

Action and mechanism: Over a period of one to two weeks of daily use, these compounds exert a gradual stimulant action on mood and appetite. They lower blood pressure, and decrease the probability of convulsions. The principal mode of action involves inactiva-

# APPENDIX I

tion of the monoamine oxidase enzymes in the brain. Antidepressants may also act directly on the synapse.

Uses: To reverse depression and melancholia and in some cases to produce extroversion in manic depressives.

Dangers: Chronic abuse causes agitation, tremor, excitement, drowsiness and dizziness. Skin diseases and other toxic effects are common. In rare cases, overdoses can even cause circulatory collapse and death.

Potential for psychological dependence: high
Potential for physiological dependence: low
Potential for tolerance: moderate

Preparations: Marsilid, Nardil, Elavil, Tofranil. Users show psychological dependence after several weeks of taking 50-100 mg daily.

## Barbiturates

Action and mechanism: Low doses depress sensory functions and produce sedation and drowsiness. High doses depress motor functions, cause confusion, and lead to sleep or anesthesia. Barbiturates are thought to interfere with the transmission of nervous information travelling toward the brain's cortex. They also enhance the activity of enzymes involved in the degradation of the body's waste products.

Uses: To produce short, intermediate, or long-term sedation, depending on the type of compound.

# APPENDIX I

<u>Dangers</u>: Overdoses cause severe depression, gloominess, and eventually coma and death by asphyxiation. Chronic abuse leads to skin diseases and confusion, or to acute anxiety and restlessness during withdrawal. Liver damage is also common.

Potential for psychological dependence: high
Potential for physiological dependence: high
Potential for tolerance: variable

<u>Preparations</u>: Seconal, Amytal, Nebutal. Daily oral doses in excess of 400 mg are sufficient to produce significant dependence.

## Belladona Alkaloids and Related Compounds

<u>Action and mechanism</u>: Cause dilation of the pupils, dry skin, mouth, and stomach; relaxation of bronchial and stomach smooth muscle. Large doses of atropine cause excitement or loss of inhibitions; scopolamine produces stronger effects than atropine, along with hallucinations or partial amnesia. These agents are thought to block uptake of acetylcholine at the synapse.

<u>Uses</u>: Atropine serves as an antispasmodic, antisecretory, or cardiac stimulant drug. Scopolamine reduces rigidity in parkinsonism. It is a sedative and pre-anesthetic medication.

<u>Dangers</u>: Overdoses cause amplification of normal effects. Fatal toxicity is rare.

# APPENDIX I

Potential for psychological dependence: low
Potential for physiological dependence: low
Potential for tolerance: not known

Preparations: Atropine, Scopolamine, Metropine, Panolid. The effective dose is approximately 0.5 mg by mouth or injection.

## Caffeine

Action and mechanism: Stimulates all parts of the nervous system to produce varying degrees of alertness, wakefulness, and talkativeness. Its mode of action at the synapse is not known, but most of its effects can be explained as a function of the drug's indirect role in promoting the enzymatic reactions necessary for enhanced energy metabolism.

Uses: To induce wakefulness.

Dangers: Overdoses produce sleeplessness and hyperactivity and an increased sensitivity to sound.

Potential for psychological dependence: moderate
Potential for physiological dependence: none
Potential for tolerance: moderate

Preparations: Coffee, tea, pills. Effective doses of pure caffeine taken by mouth are in the range of 500 to 2,000 mg daily.

# APPENDIX I

## Cocaine

*Action and mechanism:* Intermittent use causes abolition of fatigue and hunger, increased physical activity, and vivid hallucinations. Chronic use leads to toxic psychosis with compulsive, potentially anti-social acts. Cocaine depresses the sensitivity of nerve endings by elevating the threshold of nerve excitability. It apparently combines with the membranes at the synapse where it competes with neurotransmitters, primarily acetylcholine.

*Uses:* Medically, for topical anesthesia of the eye, nose, ear and throat. The attraction of cocaine as a drug of abuse lies in its use as an excitant.

*Dangers:* Overdosage produces initially a sense of pleasure, then nausea, sweating, convulsions, leading ultimately to medullary depression, cardio-vascular collapse and death.

Potential for psychological dependence: high
Potential for physiological dependence: low
Potential for tolerance: low

*Preparations:* Obtained by chewing coca leaves, or as a white powder. When injected frequently in small doses as much as 10,000 mg can be taken in one day. 100 to 300 mg intravenously produce the desired sense of excitement.

# APPENDIX I

## Inhalants

<u>Action and mechanism</u>: These volatile compounds can cause a whole spectrum of behavioral changes, ranging from mild euphoria and giggling to pronounced intoxication. They act upon the nervous system, lowering the rate of information flow out from command centers in the brain. Breathing and circulation are depressed.

<u>Uses</u>: Many are used as anesthetics in surgery. Also used in "thrills", particularly by early adolescents.

<u>Dangers</u>: Excessive use causes irreparable damage to the liver and kidneys. Single overdoses are fatal.

Potential for psychological dependence: low

Potential for physiological dependence: none

Potential for tolerance: low

<u>Preparations</u>: Ether, chloroform, nitrous oxide, volatile constituents of airplane glue, gasoline. The physiologically effective doses and concentrations are not known.

## Marihuana

<u>Action and mechanism</u>: Varying degrees of euphoria, intoxication, giggling, laughing, feeling of relief or escape, and exaggerated interpretation of objects and sensations. Mode of action unknown.

<u>Uses</u>: Social euphoriant and intoxicant.

<u>Dangers</u>: Excessive use may lead to protracted

## APPENDIX I

lethargy and indifference.

    Potential for psychological dependence: moderate
Potential for physiological dependence: low, if any
Potential for tolerance: variable

    <u>Preparations</u>: Dried plant leaves (pot), pressed resin (hashish). Effective doses are highly variable, depending on the quality of the drug preparation.

### Narcotics

    <u>Action and mechanism</u>: This broad grouping of drugs causes a combination of depression and stimulation of the nervous system; relief of pain and anxiety, relaxation of cough reflexes and muscle spasms; general sedation and mild euphoria. The mode of action is presumed to involve certain as yet undefined interactions at synapses, both deep inside the brain and in the medulla.

    <u>Uses</u>: The principal clinical use is to relieve pain. As drugs of abuse, narcotics serve to isolate users from sensory inputs and provide a feeling of intense euphoric sedation.

    <u>Dangers</u>: Acute poisoning is characterized by increasing depression, slowed respiration, pinpoint pupils, and dreamy stupor. Death results within five to ten hours after an overdose.

    Potential for psychological dependence: high

# APPENDIX I

Potential for physiological dependence: high

Potential for tolerance: high

Preparations: Opium, morphine, heroin, codeine, Dilaudid, Demerol, Percodan. An individual may begin with a dose of 2 to 8 mg, but addicts may use as much as 450 mg per day as tolerance is acquired. On the average, the user taking 40-60 mg a day (by injection) will acquire a fairly substantial habit in two weeks.

Nicotine

Action and mechanism: Action of nicotine is stimulatory, marked by increased intestinal activity; constriction of small arteries and capillaries, causing pallor, sweating, and increased blood pressure. Its mode of action resembles that of acetycholine.

Uses: Excluding tobacco smoking, too unreliable for therapeutic application in man; it is applied as a short acting anesthetic in veterinary medicine.

Dangers: Acute overdose causes respiratory arrest.

Potential for psychological dependence: high

Potential for physiological dependence: not known

Potential for tolerance: not known

Preparations: Tobacco. The effective dosage is not known.

# APPENDIX I

## Phenothiazines

Action and mechanism:  Long lasting influence in the system to reduce motor activity, induce quietness, drowsiness and apathy. Reflexes are depressed. At the level of the synapse, in general, phenothiazines block the release of neurotransmitters from storage vessels at the tips of nerve cells. They also block enzymatic reactions along various pathways toward neurotransmitter biosynthesis and metabolism. Additional mechanisms of action involve direct chemical reactions with synaptic membranes, causing reduced permeabilities.

Uses:  Most frequently prescribed as tranquilizers in the treatment of excited psychoses or of excessive nervousness.

Dangers:  Chronic use leads to weakness, chilliness, constipation, blurred vision, weight gain, and convulsions (after very high doses). May frequently cause damage to the liver and bone marrow.

Potential for psychological dependence:  moderate
Potential for physiological dependence:  low
Potential for tolerance:  low

Preparations:  Thorazine, Compazine. Effective doses vary between 10 and 200 mg two or three times a day. Psychological dependence results several weeks after continued use of approximately 500 mg a day.

# APPENDIX I

## Psychedelics (natural products)

Action and mechanism: Psychic stimulation, hallucinations, sensory amplification and distortion, visual and spatial illusions. Mode of action is highly complex and not fully understood. They are presumed to interfere primarily with neurotransmitters in the brain, particularly serotonin.

Uses: Applied as adjuncts to treatment of schizophrenia, psychosis, and alcoholism. Popular street drugs.

Dangers: Excessive doses may lead to delirium or acute (and sometimes permanent) psychosis. General after-effects may include drowsiness, dry mouth, nausea, anxiety, dizziness, and skin rashes.

Potential for psychological dependence: variable
Potential for physiological dependence: not known
Potential for tolerance: variable

Preparations: LSD, psilocybin, mescaline, DMT. The effective doses are approximately 0.1 to 0.3 mg of LSD, 300 to 400 mg of mescaline, 20 to 60 mg of psilocybin, and 50 to 60 mg of DMT.

## Psychedelics (synthetic)

Action and mechanism: Depending on the kinds of chemical groups present in their structure, these compounds produce a spectrum of effects ranging from mild

# APPENDIX I

euphoria to intense hallucinations. They are presumed to interfere chemically with the uptake and release of neurotransmitters.

Uses: Very rarely as a tool in psychotherapy. Popular street drugs.

Dangers: Excessive doses may lead to delirium or acute psychosis.

Potential for psychological dependence: variable
Potential for physiological dependence: not known
Potential for tolerance: variable

Preparations: STP, MDA, MMDA. The usual effective doses are 2 to 4 mg of STP, 150 to 250 mg of MDA, and 80 to 100 mg of MMDA.

## Reserpine Alkaloids

Action and mechanism: Low doses bring about calm, light sleep that can be easily disturbed, and diminished aggressiveness. These compounds act deep inside the brain on the hypothalamus, but the exact mode of action is still unknown.

Uses: As tranquilizers, less potent than the phenothiazines in the treatment of neurosis, psychosis, and high blood pressure.

Dangers: High doses elicit excessive sedation, nightmares, and the symptoms of Parkinson's disease. Can also cause vomiting, diarrhea, and bleeding from

# APPENDIX I

peptic ulcers.

    Potential for psychological dependence: minimal
Potential for physiological dependence: none
Potential for tolerance: low

    Preparations: Serpasil, Harmonyl, Moderil. Effective doses vary in the range of 0.1 to 0.5 mg one to three or four times a day by mouth.

## Salicylates

    Action and mechanism: Relief of pain, particularly headaches. Effective as an anti-inflammatory or anti-allergenic agent. They also stimulate respiration and cause an increase in oxygen consumption. Mode of action unknown.

    Uses: To relieve muscle and joint aches, headaches and minor infections.

    Dangers: Overdoses produce nausea, diarrhea and hallucinations. Massive overdoses can cause respiratory paralysis and death.

    Potential for psychological dependence: high
Potential for physiological dependence: low
Potential for tolerance: variable

    Preparations: Aspirin, 300 to 1,000 mg four times a day produces the desired physiological effects.

## APPENDIX I

### Sedatives

Action and mechanism: Cause varying degrees of sedation. High doses, especially of the so-called "hypnotics" cause drowsiness, vertigo and impaired thinking. The mechanism of sedation is unknown, but the mechanism of muscle relaxation is presumed to involve nerve impulse blocking reactions at synapses in the spinal cord.

Uses: Short acting tranquilizers, alternatives to barbiturates in the treatment of anxiety and tension states.

Dangers: Generally of low toxicity and overdoses are seldom fatal. Convulsion result only upon withdrawal from continued use. Some drugs in this class may also cause liver damage in chronic users.

Potential for psychological dependence: high
Potential for physiological dependence: moderate
Potential for tolerance: moderate

Preparations: Equanil, Placidyl, Librium, Valium. Large doses of Librium in the range of 300 to 600 mg a day for several months cause clinically significant symptoms of dependence. 2,400 mg a day of Equanil for a similar time period also produces dependence.

# APPENDIX II

## A Guide to Bibliographic and Literature Search Services

**Adverse Reaction Titles** (Excerpta Medica Foundation, Amsterdam) A monthly bibliography from 3,500 medical journals. Covers literature on the harmful effects of drugs.

**Biochemical Title Index** (Biological Abstracts, Inc., Philadelphia) Monthly, covering 25,000 references a year from over 500 journals worldwide. Useful as a guide to research in drug metabolism and mode of action.

**Biological Abstracts** (Biological Abstracts, Inc., Philadelphia) Monthly, comprehensive survey of biology and related fields.

**Birth Defects** (National Foundation - March of Dimes, New York) Monthly, covers 2,600 journals.

**Brain Information Center** (Brain Research Institute, University of California, Los Angeles) Literature searches primarily on neurophysiology.

**Bulletin on Narcotics** (United Nations, Geneva) Carries a quarterly bibliography to world literature on narcotics.

**Chemical Abstracts** (American Chemical Society, Washington D.C.) The most comprehensive abstracting service: 165,000 abstracts a year from over 8,000 periodicals. Collective and Decennial Indices are available.

**Chemotherapy Research Bulletin** (Chemotherapy Research

## APPENDIX II

Institute, New York) Provides information describing new drug developments in pharmacology and therapeutics.

Classified Abstract Archives of the Alcohol Literature (Rutgers Center of Alcohol Studies, New Brunswick, New Jersey) Annual, 450 abstracts of world literature on alcohol and alcoholism).

Clinical Literature Untoward Effects (CLUE) (International Information Institute, Philadelphia) Reviews of foreign literature.

John Crerar Library (Chicago, Illinois) Provides literature searches, xeroxes, and book loans. Particularly useful as a source to foreign literature on drugs since the library carries 100,000 translations and provides photocopying services.

Current Contents of Chemical Pharmacomedial and Life Sciences (Institute for Scientific Information, Philadelphia) General abstracting service of 900 journals, more than 150,000 articles worldwide.

Drug Dependence and Abuse Notes (National Clearinghouse for Mental Health Information, National Institute of Mental Health, Chevy Chase, Maryland) Annotated abstracts of literature on addiction.

Drug Digests from the Foreign Literature (National Science Foundation, Washington) Annual compilations.

Excerpta Medica (Excerpta Medica Foundation, Amsterdam) Section 2c provides monthly abstracts of international literature in pharmacology and drug toxicology.

Index Medicus (National Library of Medicine, Bethesda, Maryland) Monthly lists of article titles grouped by topic.

International Reference Center for Information on Psychotropic Drugs (Psychopharmacology Research Service Branch, National Institute of Mental Health, Chevy Chase, Maryland) Literature searches.

## APPENDIX II

<u>National Clearinghouse for Mental Health Information</u>
(National Institute of Mental Health, Chevy Chase, Maryland) Provides literature searches and publications.

<u>National Library of Medicine, Literature Searches</u> (National Library of Medicine, Bethesda, Maryland) Literature searches upon commission. Past searches are available to the public upon request.

<u>Psychological Abstracts</u> (American Psychological Association, Inc., Lancaster, Pennsylvania) Comprehensive, monthly abstracts of the international literature.

<u>Psychopharmacology Abstracts</u> (United States, Department of Health, Education and Welfare, Washington, D.C.) Abstracts of international literature. Features research reports on drug action mechanisms.

<u>Psychopharmacology Bulletin</u> (National Institute of Mental Health, Washington, D.C.) Monthly abstracts of government research reports on drugs.

<u>STASH Bibliographic Services</u> (Student Association for the Study of Hallucingoens, Inc., Beloit, Illinois) Provides literature searches, xeroxes, and book loans, particularly on subjects pertaining to hallucinogens or to marihuana.

<u>University Microfilm Library Services</u> (Ann Arbor, Michigan) Xeroxes of articles of books. This literature service is perhaps the most extensive and complete.

# SUBJECT INDEX

Note: Numbers refer to entries, not pages.

## A

Abuse of Drugs, see Drug Abuse

Acetylcholine
  biochemistry of, 3, 5, 9, 60

Addiction, see also Drug Abuse
  to alcohol, see Alcoholism
  to amphetamines, 113, 140
  to barbiturates, 126-128, 140, 142, 145
  crime and, 43, 163, 404, 410, 420, 424, 426
  definition, 43, 51, 54, 61, 156
  legal psychiatry and, 50
  to mixed drugs, 132, 140, 351
  pharmacological classifications
    and generalizations, 50, 51
  psychology of, 42, 50, 51, 150, 155, 158, 160,
    167, 170-173, 453, 480, 489
  to tranquilizers, 132, 139, 145
  treatment of, 74, 149, 153, 167, 168
  withdrawal syndromes, 73

Affective Disorder
  biochemistry of, 49, 52, 59, 168

Alcohol
  abuse of, see Alcoholism
  effects on brain metabolism, 91
  history of, 92, 283
  hangover from, 134
  toxicity of, 93, 96
  use with other drugs, 84, 90, 128, 282

Alcoholic Beverages
  effects
    on body, 86, 91

## SUBJECT INDEX

    on brain, 93, 101
    on metabolism, 93

Alcoholism
  causes of, 85, 87, 90, 94, 128
  definition of, 85, 87, 89
  physiological and psychological factors, 88, 90, 92, 97, 98
  treatment of, 83, 86, 88, 94, 95, 134

Alienation
  as motivation for drug abuse, 356, 360, 372, 394-396, 416, 418, 421

Amanita muscaria, see Fly agaric

American Indians
  peyote use by, 205, 211, 212, 216

Amines, see also Catecholamines
  brain, 15, 17, 59, 104
  Serotonin, effect of drugs on, 17, 34, 59, 65, 96

Amphetamine(s)
  abuse of, 109, 113
  addiction potential, 113, 140
  and barbiturate abuse, 103
  behavioral effects, 102, 106
  biochemical effects, 102, 106, 227, 231, 237
  classification of, 106
  clinical application of compared with cocaine, 118
  overuse symptoms, 103
  pharmacology of, 104
  toxic psychoses, 103, 109
  toxicity, 102, 113

Analgesics, see Addiction; Narcotics; Drug Abuse

Anesthetics
  effect of local, 117, 122
  narcotics as, 149

Antabuse, see Disulfiram

Antagonists, for drugs in addiction, 149, 167

Antianxiety Agents, see Tranquilizers

Antidepressants, see Stimulants

Aphrodisiacs
  drugs as, 157, 309, 430, 436, 466, 485, 491

## SUBJECT INDEX

**Art**
  drugs as stimulants for, 31, 192, 427, 433, 434, 449, 463, 477, 488, 492, 496, 508, 511, 516

**Aspirin,** see Salicylates

### B

**Barbiturates**
  addiction to, 126-128, 140, 142, 145
  death from, 127
  effect on brain metabolism, 37, 123, 124
  potential action on genes, 142
  prenatal effects, 138
  toxicology and poisoning by, 126
  use in therapy, 127, 130

**Behavior**
  control of by drugs, 58, 75, 78, 80, 82, 166, 174, 176, 195, 222
  origins of, 79, 388

**Benzedrine,** see Amphetamines

**Biogenic Amines,** see Catecholamine

**Brain**
  biochemistry, genetic variations in, 4
  cerebral energy metabolism and, 6
  definition of mind, 36
  emotional behavior and regions of, 18, 27
  metabolic effects of drugs on, 4, 17, 37
  transport reactions, effects of specific inhibitors on, 37

### C

**Caapi,** use in South America, 218, 219, 460

**Caffeine**
  pharmacology of, 60, 116, 376

**Catecholamines**
  in brain function and human behavior, 15, 16, 21, 24, 38, 49
  drug action and, 2, 25
  metabolism of, drug effects on, 21
  in schizophrenia, 52, 62

## SUBJECT INDEX

in sleep, 34

Chlordiazepoxide (Librium), see also
 Sedatives-Hypnotics
 chemistry of, 135
 pharmacology of, 147
 structure, activity and dosage, 147

Chlorpromazine (Thorazine), see also Tranquilizers
 effect,
  on central monoamine neurons, 1
  on chromosome, 146
  on memory, 131
 reaction with hallucinogens, 243

Classification of drugs, 53, 60

Clinical Pharmacology
 of drug metabolism, 60
 general principles, 63
 methodology, 46
 problems in, 56
 in treatment of drug overdoses, 167, 236, 252,
  317, 319, 328

Clinical Psychopharmacology
 methodology and problems in, 44-46, 124
 experimental design in, 46

Cocaine
 in coca leaf, 120
 effects,
  on brain metabolism, 117, 118, 122
  on cell membranes, 118

Codeine, see also Narcotics
 biochemical effects, 104

Coffee, see Caffeine

Consciousness, see also Psychopharmacological agents
 expansion of by hallucinogens, 186, 189, 203, 442,
  443, 452, 457, 486
 experience of, 29, 30, 41, 401

### D

Death, from drug use, 199, 200, 411

Death Instinct and drug use, 377, 411, 482, 489

## SUBJECT INDEX

Dexedrine, see also Amphetamine(s)
  biochemistry and chemistry of, 106, 113, 116
  effect on dreams, 37

Disulfiram (Antabuse), use in alcoholism therapy, 86

DOM, see also Hallucinogens
  as hallucinogen, 105, 107
  biochemistry and chemistry of, 112, 114, 248

Dreams
  effect of drugs on, 37, 42
  physiology of, 32, 33
  relationship to hallucination, 35

Drugs, see Psychopharmacological Agents or under individual class headings

Drug Abuse
  in sports, 340
  surveys, general, 279, 319, 332, 339, 356, 361, 372, 373, 406-408, 425, 426
  by adolescents, 331, 332, 335-337, 341, 345, 347-351, 357, 362, 365, 366, 375
  by college students, 283, 333, 343, 344, 346, 355, 358, 363
  in foreign countries, 107, 265, 336, 347, 351, 357
  by military, 344, 358, 359, 364, 367

Drug Culture, see also Psychopharmacological Agents; Youth Culture
    studies on, 356, 360, 372, 373, 375, 378, 383, 384, 386, 391, 393, 400, 409, 419, 425, 448, 450, 453, 455, 462, 471, 481, 495, 507, 526

Drug Industry
  social responsibility of, 399, 408, 413, 420, 425, 453

Drug Research
  ethical design in, 47, 67, 371, 387, 420
  on children, 70
  on mental patients, 77

E

Emotions, see Behavior
  chemistry of, 38, 40

Ether, used in mind expansion, 445

Extrasensory Perception (ESP), use of drugs in, 185, 189

## SUBJECT INDEX

### F

Fly Agaric (Soma)
  ethnopsychopharmacology of, 3, 55, 217, 224, 225

### G

Genes
  effect of drugs on, 138, 142, 165, 228, 230, 234

Glue Sniffing, see Inhalants

### H

Haight-Ashbury
  drug culture in, 107, 278, 288, 381, 385, 413

Hallucinations
  causes of, 30, 41, 42, 109, 520, 521
  relationship to dreams, 35, 428, 438, 465

Hallucinogens, see also individual categories
  abuse of, 253, 346, 352
  chemistry and biochemistry of, 207, 218-220, 232, 235, 240, 241, 255, 257, 259, 260
  complications, 199, 250, 253
  description of effects of, 201, 204
  general information about, 180, 194, 214, 223
  treatment of bad trips, 167, 317, 319, 328

Hedonism
  drugs as force in, 373, 383

Heroin, see also Addiction; Opiates
  in adolescents, 151, 162
  impressionistic description of effects, 150, 160, 178, 440, 447, 470, 499
  initial causes for use of, 171-173
  narcotic antagonists, 149, 156, 175
  postwithdrawal treatment, 153
  in urban communities, 163

Histamine
  in brain, 1, 14

Hippie Culture
  effect of drugs in, 338, 377, 378, 382, 389, 391

## SUBJECT INDEX

Hypnosis
  hallucinogens as agents in, 193, 431, 452

### I

Inhalants
  effects of, 305, 306, 308-313
  toxicity of, 307

Insanity, see Psychosis

### J

Jesus
  as symbol in drug culture, 429, 481

### L

Librium, see Chlordiazepoxide

Literature
  drugs as motivation in, 427, 433, 434, 447, 449, 463, 516

Love
  as theme in drug culture, 379, 435

Lysergic acid diethylamide (LSD)
  abuse of, 184, 186, 196, 235, 251, 367
  biochemistry of, 188, 231, 237, 249, 252
  clinical test on, 245
  complications, including genetic, 199, 201, 228, 234, 239, 246, 247, 250, 262-264
  effect on dreams, 42, 243
  effect on speech, 182, 197
  hallucinogenic action mechanism, 14, 20, 226
  history of, 180, 181, 190, 244
  metabolism of, 229
  pharmacology, comparative, 20
  psychic and psychotherapeutic effects, 59, 83, 179, 181, 185, 186, 189, 195, 202, 203, 254, 431, 486
  reaction with tranquilizers, 243
  treatment of, 236, 252, 317, 319, 328
  in treatment of alcoholism, 59, 83, 94, 187

# SUBJECT INDEX

## M

Marihuana
  adverse effects of, 267, 294
  abuse of, legal aspects of, 277, 285
  biochemistry and chemistry of, 226, 293, 295-304,
  comparison to effects of alcohol, 282, 283
  ethnopharmacology of, 266, 269, 270, 275, 276, 278-281,
    286-288, 290, 292, 373, 431
  pharmacology of, 265, 268, 271-274, 284, 289

MDA
  abuse of, 107, 108, 112
  biochemistry and chemistry, 248

Memory
  chemistry of, 36, 39
  effect of tranquilizers on, 132, 148

Mental Disease
  nature of, 19

Mescaline
  as active principle in peyote, 208
  biochemistry and chemistry, 208, 231, 233, 238, 245,
    252, 258
  compared with TMA, 110, 112
  genetic complications, 233, 239
  as hallucinogen, 210, 245, 261

Methadone
  addiction to, 152
  in addiction therapy, 153, 175, 390, 403

Monoamine Oxidase Inhibitors, 21

Morphine, see also Heroin; Addiction
  addiction to, 152, 155, 158, 162
  chemistry of, 149, 161, 164, 169

Mushrooms, hallucinogenic, see Peyote; Psilocybin; Fly Agaric

Mysticism
  drugs as influence in, 467, 468, 471, 473, 475, 502,
    503, 505, 513, 524, 525, 527

# SUBJECT INDEX

## N

Narcotics, see individual listings
  addiction to, 168
  classification, 149

Nerve Endings, 11, 12

**Neurons**
  central monoamine type, 11, 12
  characteristics of, 15

Nicotine
  effects, 60

**Nutmeg**
  ethnopharmacology, 55, 60, 218, 219

## O

Opiates, see Addiction, Heroin, Morphine
  addiction to, 154, 155, 157
  chemistry of, 60, 75, 149, 164
  effect on behavior, 166

Opium
  effect on dreams, 42, 447, 458, 463
  history of, 57, 69, 154, 159, 441, 447, 528

## P

Pain
  effect of analgesics on, 44, 133
  measurement of, 44-47, 124

Pediatric Psychopharmacology, 69, 151, 250

Perception
  relationship to hallucination, 30, 203, 434, 437, 456, 457, 464, 510

Peyote, see also Mescaline
  chemistry of, 206-208
  as religion, 205, 211, 212, 216, 221

Phenothiazines, see also Tranquilizers
  addiction to, 132

# SUBJECT INDEX

chemistry of, 125
effect on childbirth, 138

Placebo
in drug tests, 44-47

Prenatal Drug Administration, 132, 165

Prognostic scales, in drug evaluation, 60

Protocols for drug research, design, 46, 60

Psilocybin, see also Hallucinogens
chemistry of, 218, 219
as hallucinogen, 202, 209, 213-215, 222, 245

Psychedelics, see Hallucinogens

Psychopharmacological Agents
abuse of, see Drug Abuse, Addiction
chemistry of, 4, 7, 10, 53, 60, 64, 66, 71, 75
chemical identification and diagnosis of, 58, 314-330
in creativity and art, 31, 192, 427, 433, 434, 449,
  463, 477, 488, 492, 496, 508, 511, 516
dosage of, 60, 71
ethnopharmacology of, general, 55, 56, 69
evaluation techniques, 44-46, 56, 68, 72, 76
federal regulations on, 72, 399, 424
history of, 60, 66, 67, 69, 410, 425, 455, 507
in imagination and ecstasy, 28, 432, 433, 434, 437,
  445, 451, 456, 457, 460, 471, 493, 496, 497, 519
law and, 66, 369, 390, 397, 404, 410, 412, 424, 426,
  469
molecular receptor of, theory of, 8, 23, 39
in mysticism, 467, 468, 471, 473, 475, 502, 503, 505,
  513, 524, 525, 527
in religion, 429, 439, 442-444, 446, 459, 474, 479,
  481, 483, 484, 494, 512
research on, controversial issues, 47, 67, 371, 399,
  420
sensory and perceptual processes and, 44-46
sorcery and, 459, 528, 529
in study design with humans and animals, 7, 21, 46, 47,
  56, 78
terminology in descriptions of, 53, 60, 76
therapy using, 73, 77, 81, 83, 423
value to society, 230, 370-373, 375, 376, 379, 380, 408,
  413, 420, 425, 448, 461, 471, 486, 507, 515

Psychosis, 13, 29, 428, 438, 464, 465, 476, 489

## SUBJECT INDEX

### R

Religion
  drugs as part of ritual in, 429, 439, 442-444, 446, 459, 479, 481, 484, 494, 512, 528

Reserpine (Serpasil)
  addiction to, 132
  in catecholamine function, 1
  chemistry of, 60, 141
  prenatal effects of, 138

Rock music
  drug oriented lyrics in, 469, 515

### S

Salicylates
  chemistry of, 129, 137
  as enzyme inhibitors, 136

Schizophrenia, see also Psychosis
  biochemical mechanism of, 48, 62, 65, 261
  description of, 465

Sedatives-Hypnotics
  biochemistry and chemistry of, 130, 147
  effect on dreams, 37

Sensory Processes, 26, 27, 30

Sernyl (Phenocyclidine)
  as hallucinogen, 183, 198, 202

Serotonin, see Amines

Sex, see Aphrodisiacs

Sleep, mechanisms for, 32-34

Snuff, Hallucinogenic, of South America, 55, 218, 219

Social Control
  drugs as agents in, 369, 390, 403, 412, 422, 495

Soma, see Fly Agaric

South America
  coca leaf use in, 120, 121, 218
  hallucinogenic snuffs of, 55

## SUBJECT INDEX

Speech
  brain function in, 20

Stimulants, see also individual listings
  abuse of, 113
  classification of, 53, 60
  effect on dreams, 42
  mode of action, 115

STP, see DOM

Synapse
  chemically transmitting, 5, 9

Synaptic junctions
  receptors at, 8, 257

## T

Tea, ethnopharmacology of, 101, 376

Therapy, using psychopharmacologic agents,
  see also individual listings, 77, 81, 83, 94, 95,
  127, 130, 134, 149, 153

Tobacco
  addiction to, 348
  psychopharmacology, 90, 99, 376

Tranquilizers, see also individual listings
  classification and chemistry of, 124, 130, 141
  effect on newborn, 138
  use to treat hangovers, 134

## W

Witchcraft
  drugs in, 459, 475, 528, 529

## Y

Youth Culture, see Drug Abuse, Drug Culture, Hippies

# AUTHOR INDEX

Aaronson, B.S., 179, 180
Abbey, H., 350
Aberle, D.F., 205
Abrams, M.H., 427
Abramson, H.A., 83, 197
Adam, H.M., 1
Adams, E., 123
Adams, J.K., 428
Adams, R.L., 429
Adams, W.T., 306
Addiction Research Foundation, 84
Adler, N., 370
Adrian, E.D., 26
Adriani, J., 149
Advisory Committee on Drug Dependence, 265
Agar, M.A., 177
Aghajamian, G.K., 226, 237
Agnew, D., 369
Alexander, M., 430
Allen, J.R., 278
Alpert, R., 181, 401, 482

Amarel, M., 182
Amini, F., 183
Andrews, G., 266
Anglert, L.F., 297
Antun, F., 227, 256
Anumonye, A., 331
Ariani, J., 117
Asbey, H., 365
Auerbach, R., 228
Austin, B.L., 150
Ausubel, D.P., 43
Axelrod, J., 2, 229, 296

Baker, R.W., 3
Bakker, C.B., 183
Baldridge, B.J., 42
Barber, B., 371
Barber, T.X., 431
Barfknecht, C.F., 227
Barker, G.H., 306
Barron, F., 432
Barter, J.T., 353
Baudelaire, C., 433

## AUTHOR INDEX

Bays, G., 434

Bearg, R.D., 305

Beecher, H.K., 44, 45, 46, 47, 124, 152, 162, 174

Bejerot, N., 118

Belmann, S.W., 314

Bender, L., 230

Benington, F., 227, 258

Bergman, R.L., 206

Bewley, T.H., 372

Bialos, D.S., 267

Bishop, M.G., 435

Black, P., 4

Black, S., 332

Bleibtraub, J.N., 373

Blewett, D.B., 185

Bloch, I., 436

Blood, B.P., 437

Bloom, F.E., 5

Bloomquist, E.R., 268

Blos, P., 374

Blum, J., 375

Blum, R.H., 376

Blyer-Prieto, H., 119

Boethals, G.W., 363

Boisen, A., 438

Boueton, A.A., 48

Bouthilet, L., 68

Bowen, H.L., 362

Boyd, J.E., 85

Boyd, P., 151

Braden, W., 439

Bradley, D.W., 102

Bradley, P.B., 6, 125

Bradley, R.J., 79, 258

Brady, R.O., 229

Brandkamp, W.W., 247

Brickman, H.R., 377

Brill, H., 366

Brotmas, R., 333

Brown, J.D., 378

Brown, N.O., 379

Browning, E., 307

Bryson, G., 49

Budini, R., 231

Bunnell, S., 110

Burnett, G.B., 86

Burn-Gulbrandsen, S., 347

Burroughs, W., 440, 460

Burton, R., 441

Butler, W.P., 320

Byer, C.O., 90

Byrd, O.E., 50

Byrne, U.P., 94

## AUTHOR INDEX

Caldwell, W.V., 187
Canadian Government Commission of Inquiry, 64
Carey, J.J., 334
Carson, D.I., 335
Carstairs, G.M., 269
Casteneda, C., 442
Castaneda, C., 443
Cavanna, R., 189
Chambers, C.D., 126
Charbonneau, L., 380
Cheek, F.E., 182, 315
Chopra, R.N., 270
Chothia, C.H., 3, 232
Chow, K.L., 27
Clark, L.C., 258
Clark, L.D., 291
Clark, W.G., 7
Clark, W.H., 444
Clinco, A.A., 313
Cohen, H., 336
Cohen, M., 337
Cohen, S., 181, 352
Collier, H.D., 51
Conney, A.H., 127
Conwell, P.H., 103
Coppen, A., 52
Cornell, J.M., 147

Cutting, W.C., 53

Dalton, D., 382
Daly, C.D., 308
d'Arconte, L., 318
Datta, R.K., 233
Davidow, B., 316
Davie, J.S., 346
Davis, F., 338
Davy, H., 445
Davydova, O.N., 295
Debold, R.C., 190
De Felice, P., 446
De Gross, J., 317
del Giudice, J., 7
Denton, J.E., 152
Denusch, L., 24
De Quincey, T., 447
de Rench, V.S., 78
De Robertis, E., 8
De Ropp, R.S., 448
Devenyi, P., 128
Dharir, H.I., 329
Didion, J., 381
Dimijian, G.C., 319
Dishotsky, N.I., 234
Dixon, A. St. J., 129
Dole, V.P., 153

## AUTHOR INDEX

Domino, E.F., 130
Done, A.K., 311
Donnelly, H., 349
Doty, B.A., 131
Doty, L.A., 131
Drug Abuse Project Report to the Ford Foundation, 339
Duane, B., 316
Durr, R.A., 449

Ebin, D., 450
Eccles, J., 9, 28, 29
Eddy, N.B., 54
Eells, K., 191
Efron, D.H., 55, 56
Egozcue, J., 246
Eliade, M., 451
Elkes, J., 6
Ellis, E.S., 57
Encyclopedia Britannica, 154
Epstein, L.J., 402, 403
Erikson, M.H., 452
Essig, C.F., 132
Evarts, E.V., 229, 235

Fabing, H.D., 236
Fadiman, J., 192
Faillace, L., 114
Farber, L.H., 453

Farnsworth, N.R., 207
Farnsworth, D., 454
Fayez, M.B.E., 208
Felton, D., 382
Finlator, J., 455
Fischer, R., 30, 456, 457, 508
Fitzherbert, J., 309
Fogel, S., 193
Folch, Pi., J., 10
Foote, W.E., 226, 237
Formanek, J., 243
Forney, R.B., 329, 330
Fort, J., 58, 383
Fox, A.M., 392
Fox, R.J., 429
Fraser, H.F., 139, 155
Freedman, D.X., 240, 293
Friedhoff, A.J., 238
Fritchie, G.E., 297
Fron, D.H., 135
Fuller, J.G., 458
Furst, P.T., 459

Galambos, E., 104
Galambos, R., 11
Gamage, J.R., 271
Gardner, E., 12

## AUTHOR INDEX

Gardener, H., 384
Gates, M., 133
Geber, W.F., 239
Ghosh, J.J., 233
Giarman, N.J., 240
Gibbins, R.J., 140
Gilbert, B., 340
Gillespie, H.K., 299, 230
Gilman, A., 60
Ginsberg, A., 460
Gitchoff, G.T., 341
Glassman, A., 59
Gloscia, V., 385
Gloye, E.E., 241
Goaf, W., 283
Goethals, G.W., 342
Goldberg, L., 134
Goldberg, M.E., 135
Goldstein, A., 156
Goldstein, L., 13
Golightly, B.H., 514
Goode, E., 272, 292, 343
Goodman, L.S., 60
Goodwin, D., 87
Gordon, N., 386
Gorss, M., 137
Gottheif, T., 31

Gotz, I.L., 461
Gramer-Doyeux, M., 120
Greder, J.F., 344
Green, J.P., 14, 15, 258
Green, W.J., 242
Greenberg, L.A., 137
Greiner, T., 387
Grinspoon, L., 273, 274
Grisolia, S., 136
Gunn, J.W., 320
Gustaitis, R., 462
Guttman, E., 488
Guyton, A.C., 16
Gyorgy, L., 104

Halaz, M.F., 243
Hall, E.T., 388
Hammer, G.G., 198
Hanna, J.M., 121
Harman, W.W., 192
Harris, R.T., 61
Harrison, A., 519
Hartman, A.M., 245
Headlee, R., 464
Heinlein, R.A., 389
Hennell, T., 465
Herbert, C.C., 40

## AUTHOR INDEX

Herz, S., 466
Herzog, E., 345
Hesse, E., 157
Hesse, H., 467, 468
Hessling, R., 198
Heyman, F., 390
Himwich, H.E., 17, 62, 252
Himwich, W.A., 17
Hixson, J.R., 367
Ho, B.T., 297
Hoffeld, D.R., 138
Hoffer, A., 63, 88, 193, 194
Hoffman, A., 391
Hoffman, F.G., 75
Hofmann, A., 220, 244
Hollander, L., 469
Hollister, L., 114
Hollister, L.E., 105, 245, 275, 300
Hollister, L.F., 299
Holmstedt, B., 198
Holtzman, D., 293
Horman, R.E., 392
Houston, J., 492, 493
Hubbard, A.M., 94
Hughes, H.M., 470
Hughes, R., 291
Huxley, A., 393, 471, 519

Huxley, J., 472
Hyater, A., 463
Hye, H.K.A., 1

Idapaan-Heikkita, J.E., 297
Imperi, L.L., 346
Irgens-Jensen, O., 347
Irwin, S., 246
Isbell, H., 139, 155
Israel, Y., 89
Itil, T.M., 32
Iversen, L.L., 5

Jacobs, M.A., 348
Jaffe, J.H., 293
James, W., 473, 474
Jamison, K., 281
Jarvik, M.E., 197
Jenney, E.H., 13
Joffe, M., 315
Johnson, C.E., 475
Johnson, D.W., 320
Johnson, K.G., 349, 350, 365
Johnston, U.S., 79, 258
Jones, K., 90
Jones, R.T., 184
Jouvet, M., 33, 34
Joyce, D., 102
Judd, L.L., 247

## AUTHOR INDEX

Kahn, H., 412
Kaitstha, K.K., 321
Kalant, H., 140
Kalyanpur, S.G., 122
Kaminstein, P., 361
Kang, S., 248
Kapadia, G.J., 208
Kaplan, B., 476
Kaplan, J., 276, 277
Kass, W., 35
Katsiaficas, M.D., 323
Kaufman, J., 278
Keeler, M.H., 209
Kehoe, M.J., 141
Keller, R.A., 322
Keniston, K., 394, 396
Kety, S.S., 39, 62, 65
Keup, W., 294
Key, G.J., 249
Kielholz, P., 91
King, F.W., 279
King, L.J., 330
Kleber, H.D., 346
Klee, G., 195
Klein, D.F., 337
Klos, S., 342
Kluver, H., 210

Knights, J., 78
Kobler, J., 196
Kolb, L., 158
Kopin, I., 296
Kornetsky, C., 250
Kramer, M., 42
Kram, T.C., 314
Krantz, S., 397
Kris, E., 477
Kritikos, P.G., 159
Kudrin, A.N., 295
Kupperstein, L.R., 310
Kurland, A., 81
Kyogoku, Y., 142

La Barre, W., 211, 212, 478
Laing, R.D., 398, 479
Larner, J., 160
Lasagna, L., 143, 161, 162, 174, 399
Latendresse, J., 480
Laties, V.G., 116
Laurie, P., 66
Leaf, R.C., 190
Leake, C.D., 67, 106
Leary, T., 400, 401, 481, 482, 483, 484, 498, 523
Leary, T.R., 213
LeBlanc, A.E., 140

## AUTHOR INDEX

Leiderman, P.H., 144
Leihy, R., 81
Leinman, A.L., 27
Leinwald, G., 407
Lemberg, L., 296
Lennard, H., 197, 402
Lennard, H.L., 403
Leride, J., 68
Lerner, M., 323
Lewin, L., 69
Lewis, B., 485
Lewis, J.M., 335
Lieber, C., 98
Lilly, J.C., 486
Lindesmith, A.R., 404
Lindgren, J.E., 198
Lingeman, R.R., 71
Lipscomb, W.R., 234
Litwin, G.H., 213, 215
Loiselle, P., 351
Longham, W.D., 234
Lord, R.C., 142
Louria, D.B., 405, 406
Loveel, R.A., 293
Lucia, S., 92
Lundquist, F., 93
Luria, A.R., 18

Lystad, M.H., 487
McCabe, O., 81
McClure, J.L., 331
McConnell, H.M., 146
MacDonald, D.C., 94
McGeer, P.L., 36
McGlothlin, W.H., 214, 247, 281, 352, 495
McIsaac, W.M., 61, 297
McKim, R.H., 192
McNew, J., 138
McWhinne, H.J., 496
Maclay, W.S., 488
MacLean, J.R., 94
Manian, A.A., 135
Marcus, R.J., 241
Mardones, J., 89
Marinangeli, A., 231
Maris, R.W., 489
Marrazzi, A.S., 243
Marsh, R.P., 490
Martin, B.K., 129
Martin, W.R., 155
Masters, R.E.L., 491, 492, 493
Maupin, E.W., 494
Maurer, J.I., 328
Mayor's Committee on Marihuana, 280

## AUTHOR INDEX

Mechoulam, R., 298
Melges, F.T., 299, 300
Mendelson, J., 136, 144
Merril, C.R., 260
Metzner, R., 213, 215, 482, 497, 498, 523
Meyer, R.E., 199
Meyers, F.H., 107
Milbauer, B., 407
Miller, J.G., 80
Miller, J., 238
Mills, J., 499
Mintz, M., 408
Mizner, G.L., 353
Modell, W., 72
Mogar, R.E., 192, 234, 500
Molmar, J., 104
Moreau, J., 501
Morgan, D.W., 344
Morin, R.D., 258
Moscow, A., 163
Moun, R.D., 227
Munoz, L., 338
Murphree, H.B., 13
Murphy, E.H., 102

Nakashima, E.N., 291
Naranjo, D., 108, 113

Nash, B.M., 102
National Institute of Mental Health, 70
National Library of Medicine Literature Searches, 73, 74, 95, 200, 201, 301, 302, 410, 411
National Research Council, 164
Nelsen, J.M., 304
Neuberg, R., 165
Neumeyer, J.L., 303
Newell, S., 315
Newitt, J., 412
Nichols, D.E., 227
Nichols, J.R., 166
Niyogi, S.K., 324
Noguera, R., 52
Norton, P.R.E., 145
Nowlis, H.H., 354
Nyswander, M., 153

Onishi, S.I., 146
Orcutt, J.D., 282
Ornstein, P.H., 42
Osmond, H., 63, 88, 180, 194
Oswald, I., 37
Ouspensky, P.D., 502
Ownes, K.L., 332

## AUTHOR INDEX

Palaic, D., 96
Palfai, T., 147
Papdaki, S.P., 159
Pauling, L., 19
Pauling, P., 3, 232
Penfield, W., 20
Penner, W., 503
Pennington, W., 216
Petcher, T.J., 3
Pfefferbaum, D., 184
Pfeifer, A.L., 104
Pfeiffer, C.C., 13
Pharmacology Society Symposium, 167
Phillips, A.F., 355
Pierce, C.M., 263
Pietri, N. Li, 316
Plato, 504
Pollard, J.C., 202
Pope, G., 356
Pope, H.G., 363
Porsoet, R.D., 102
Prange, A.J., 52
Press, E., 311
Prince, R., 505
Proger, S., 413
Psychedelic Review, eds., 414, 506

Pscheidt, G.R., 21
Puharich, A., 217
Purpura, D.P., 22
Ramachandran, S., 330
Ramirez, E., 168
Randall, L.O., 169
Rand, M.E., 283
Rang, H.P., 23
Ranson, D.C., 402
Ray, O.S., 507
Reinhardt, C.F., 312
Reynolds, A.K., 169
Richelson, E., 259
Rich, H., 142
Rinaldi, F., 252
Roberts, L., 20
Robertson, J.A., 426
Rockney, M., 508
Root, W.S., 75
Rose, A.J., 107
Roseman, B., 509
Rosenblatt, S., 281
Rosenthal, M.S., 403
Rosenthal, S.N., 253
Rosevear, J., 284
Roszak, T., 415
Roueche, B., 97

## AUTHOR INDEX

Rubin, E., 98
Rugowski, J.A., 228
Russell, M.A., 99
Russo, J.R., 109
Ryman, B.E., 122

Santos, I., 136
Sargent, T., 108, 110, 113
Sauri, J.J., 510
Savage, C., 81, 505
Scheble, R., 349, 350
Schele, R., 365
Schiele, B.C., 68
Schildkraut, J.J., 38
Schmitt, F.O., 5, 39
Schneider, H., 24
Schultes, R.E., 218, 219, 220
Schuster, D.R., 61
Schwartz, B.N., 511
Schwartz, M., 325
Schweitzer, J.W., 238
Scott, J.M., 100
Seiler, N., 24
Select Committee on Crime, 285
Serafetinides, H., 254
Servadis, E., 189
Shaffer, I., 81

Shagowry, R.A., 303
Shainberg, L.W., 90
Sheard, M.H., 226, 237
Sheehy, G., 416
Shepherd, M., 76
Shock, H., 81
Shulgin, A.T., 108, 110, 111, 113
Silberstein, S.D., 296
Silva, J.A.F. de, 318
Silverman, I., 333
Silverman, J., 255
Simmons, J.L., 286, 417
Simon, A., 40
Simon, J., 326
Singer, M., 412
Sivasankar, D.V., 230
Slater, P., 418
Slotkin, J., 221
Smart, R.G., 357
Smith, B.C., 358
Smith, D.E., 107, 113, 288
Smith, H., 512
Smith, J., 375
Smith, J.P., 366
Smith, M.J.H., 129
Smythies, J.R., 25, 62, 79, 227, 256, 257, 258

## AUTHOR INDEX

Snyder, S.H., 114, 259, 260
Sohn, D., 326
Solomon, D., 203, 287
Solomon, P., 77, 144
Spilken, A.Z., 348
Stace, W.T., 513
Stafford, P., 419, 514
Stanton, M.D., 359
Stearn, J., 360
Steinberg, H., 78, 170
Stein, H., 402
Sterglanz, H., 264
Stern, E., 202
Sternbach, L.H., 148
Stockings, G.T., 261
Stolaroff, M.J., 192
Stone, G.C., 184
Straus, R., 40
Suffet, F., 333
Sugarman, H.A., 13
Summerfield, A., 102
Sunshine, I., 327
Sussman, R.M., 310

Talalay, P., 420
Tannebaum, A., 421
Taqi, S., 515, 516
Tart, G.T., 41, 289

Taylor, R., 517
Taylor, R.L., 328
Tefferteller, R., 160
Tewari, S., 101
Thomas, W.D., 263
Thurlow, C., 283
Tinklenberg, J.R., 299, 300, 328
Torgo, R., 361
Turczan, J.W., 314
Turk, R.F., 329, 330
Twyman, W.A., 102

Uhr, L., 80, 202
Ungerleider, J.T., 362
Unger, S., 81
Unger, S.M., 222
United States Public Health Service, 204

Vaillant, G.E., 171, 172, 173
Van Horn, G.D., 155
Van Kaam, A., 518
Van Rossum, J.M., 115
Vinkenoog, S., 266
Vlacker, K.H., 184
Von Felsinger, J.M., 162, 174

Wagner, T.E., 262
Wakefield, D., 519

## AUTHOR INDEX

Walsh, J., 175, 422
Walters, P., 363
Walton, R.P., 290
Wasson, R.G., 223, 224, 225
Wasson, V.P., 225
Watts, A.W., 423, 520, 521
Wayne, G.G., 313
Webster, R.L., 138
Weeks, J.R., 176
Weil, A.T., 304, 364, 522
Weil, G.M., 215, 523
Weiss, B., 116
Weitman, M., 349, 350, 365
Wentz-Evans, W., 524
Weppuer, R.S., 177
Werme, P.H., 353
Westhues, K., 525
West, L.J., 263, 278
Wexler, D., 144
Whitehead, P.C., 351
White, R., 308
Whitman, R.M., 42
Whybrow, P.C., 52
Wine, R.L., 349
Winograd, B., 417
Witkop, B., 229
Wittenborn, J.R., 366

Wittenborn, S.A., 366
Wolbach, A.B., 155
Wolfe, T., 526
Wolff, R.P., 332
Wolf, S., 81
Wolstenholme, G.E., 82
Wood, P.H.N., 129
Woods, R.W., 424

Yablonsky, L., 178
Yielding, K.L., 264
Young, J.H., 425
Young, W.R., 367

Zaehner, R.C., 527
Zerkin, E.L., 271
Zilboorg, G., 528, 529
Zinberg, N.E., 304, 368, 426